MANUAL OF PRACTICAL PHYSIOLOGY

Edited by
Dr Varun Malhotra
MD, DNB, NDDY
Professor, Department of Physiology
Santosh Medical College
Ghaziabad, U.P. (India)
Formerly Professor and HOD
Department of Physiology
Vinayaka Mission's Medical College
Salem, Tamil Nadu (India)

and

Dr O P Tandon
MD, MNAMS, FIABS, FAMS
Ex-Principal, Professor and Head
Department of Physiology
UCMS and GTB Hospital, Delhi (India)

PEEPEE
PUBLISHERS AND DISTRIBUTORS (P) LTD.

Manual of Practical Physiology

Published by
Pawaninder P. Vij

Peepee Publishers and Distributors (P) Ltd.
Head Office: 160, Shakti Vihar, Pitam Pura, Delhi-110 034 (India)

Correspondence Address:
7/31, First Floor, Ansari Road, Daryaganj
New Delhi-110 002 (India)
Ph: 65195868, 9811156083, 23246245
e-mail: peepee160@yahoo.co.in
e-mail: peepee160@rediffmail.com
e-mail: peepee160@gmail.com
www.peepeepub.com

First Edition: **2012**

ISBN: 978-81-8445-114-6

Printed by :
BALAJI OFFSET PRINTERS, New Delhi-110035

"Guru Brahma Guru Vishnu Guru Deva Maheshvarah;
Guru Sakshat Parabrahma Tasmeh Sri Guruveh Namah"

There is no known comparison in all three worlds for the venerable teacher that bestows knowledge. If the philosopher's stone be assumed as such, it only turns iron into gold, but alas! cannot convert it into philosopher's stone. The venerable teacher, on the other hand, creates equality with himself in the disciple that takes refuge in his feet. He is therefore peerless, nay and even transcendental.

This book is dedicated to the lotus feet of Agastya rishi, Bhagvan Krishna, Lord Jesus Christ, Mahavtar Babaji, Sri Lahiri Mahasaya, Swamy Sri Yukteshvarji and beloved Gurudeva Paramhansa Yoganandji.

Varun Malhotra

Preface

This book has been written to help the postgraduate and MBBS students in learning Physiology practicals and in maintaining a record of their observations. This would serve as a quick revision during preparations for exams. The need is felt as there is no standardized record for students in our medical colleges. A standardized record has been designed in line with the new curriculum policy of Medical Council of India. This record shall bring about uniformity in all medical colleges for practicals in Physiology.

The objectives include:

1. To inculcate the habit of inquiry in students by asking questions as to why they want to do particular experiment.
2. To develop skills using precise instruments and techniques.
3. Make use of their senses like seeing, touching (palpation), hearing (auscultation) and tapping (percussion) during examination of human organ systems.
4. Ultimate aim is to elicit and prove the authenticity of particular well-established technique, concept or physiological phenomenon.
5. Think about the application of the experiment done and its clinical use.
6. Do and learn interactive method of learning for the students in the laboratory.

Authors wish to acknowledge Dr Neelima, Dr Neelam Vaney, Dr S Sircar, Dr Savita Singh, Dr Pratibha Gupta for their help and support from time to time and also Dr Radha Krishna, for his valuable suggestions and professional help.

Our heartfelt gratitude to Pawaninder Pal Vij, Director, Peepee Publishers and Distributors (P) Ltd. for bringing out our book.

Our best wishes to all the readers and aspirants to make use of the record book.

Authors

Acknowledgements

I wish to profusely thank and acknowledge with all sincerity.

Dr (Mrs) Monica Malhotra, my wife, philosopher and guide who is a constant source of inspiration.

Mr GK Malhotra, who with his vast experience, maturity and knowledge is always there to guide in times of need. His macrolevel view and fatherly figure approach cleared many a doubt and removed the cobwebs. His pains taking efforts and invaluable suggestions helped overcome cringed situations and iron out my problems. His pleasing mannerism, cool temperament and ever smiling face is always reassuring and a source of monumental strength.

Dr. (Mrs) Kamal Malhotra, who is willing to listen and give the most apt advice during the most intricate problems and help overcome indecisive scenarios. She is a moral booster and inspirational force.

I am indebted forever to my parents for educating and inspiring me towards higher academic pursuits.

Jai Ganga and Dr Sivagami students who assisted in drafting portions of the book.

Varun Malhotra

Contents

PART - I
BLOOD

PART - II
HUMAN EXPERIMENTS

PART - I

BLOOD

1 INTRODUCTION TO HAEMATOLOGY PRACTICALS

Haematology practicals cover the experiments on blood and include haemoglobin, red blood cell count, total and differential leucocyte count, reticulocyte and platelet count, blood groups, bleeding and clotting time, packed cell volume and erythrocyte sedimentation rate etc. These investigations have direct clinical importance.

For carrying out the routine haematological work, following minimum items are needed and a preliminary knowledge of these requisites is necessary.

- Compound microscope.
- Blood sample.
- Anticoagulants.
- Different diluting fluids.
- Glass slides, pipettes and counting chambers.

COMPOUND MICROSCOPE AND ITS USE

The compound microscope is an optical instrument employing a system of lenses to magnify any object, which is ordinarily not visible to the naked eye. Except some investigation like ESR, PCV, Hb, we need the microscope for the other experiments. There are two types of microscope–monocular and binocular.

Parts of a Compound Microscope

1. **Base:** This provides stability to the instrument.
2. **Limb:** It bears:

a. *A Mechanical Stage:* Which is a platform for placing the slides containing the object. The stage has a round aperture in its center and rack and pinion mechanism for moving the slide both in antero-posterior and lateral directions.

b. *A Sub-Stage* consisting of:

i. *Condenser:* This is an assembly of lenses and it converges and concentrates the rays on the object. It can be raised or lowered with a screw.

ii. *Iris Diaphragm:* This helps in regulating the amount of light.

iii. *Filter:* This allows the monochromatic light to pass.

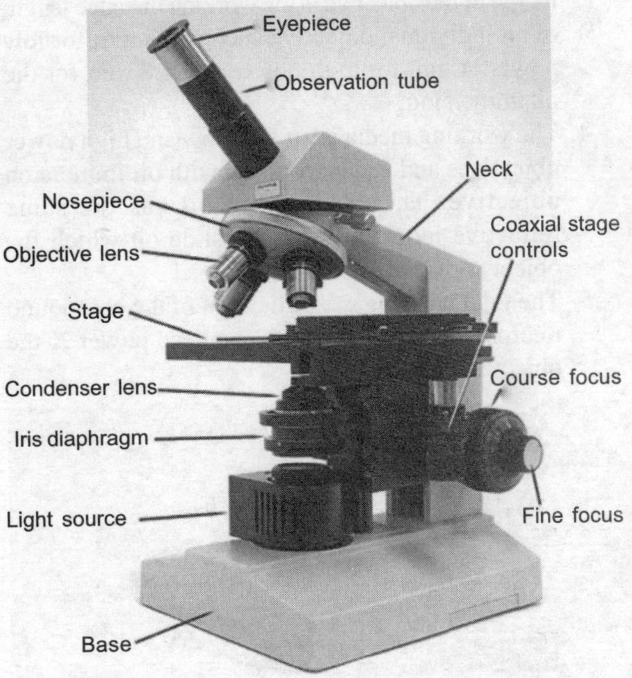

Fig. 1.1

iv. *Mirrors:* Two types of mirrors are provided: a plane one and a concave one. The mirrors reflect the light from a source of illumination through the condenser on the surface of the object.

3. **Body:** This can be divided into:

a. *The Body Proper:* This houses a coarse and a fine focussing adjustment, which is operated by, milled heads. The coarse adjustments are for moving the body tube and the fine adjustment for clarity of the image of the object.

b. *The Body Tube:*

1. This has an upper part carrying the eyepiece and a lower part carrying a revolving nosepiece or objective, which has three types of objective lenses namely low power, high power and oil immersion.
2. The eyepieces are of different powers like 5X, 6X, 10X or 15X, engraved on the eyepiece. In the

eyepiece, a vertical magnified inverted image of the object is formed.

3. The desired objective lens is placed closed to object on the stage and it produces a real, magnified and inverted primary image. The magnifications of these objectives are 10, 40 and 100 times respectively and are engraved on the objective. The magnification of the objective can be calculated by the formula.

$$\frac{\text{Mechanical tube length}}{\text{Focal length of the objective}}$$

The mechanical length of the tube is the distance between the upper part of objective and the eyepiece. It varies from 160-170 mm. The focal length of the objective is the working distance length of an individual objective such as 16 mm for low power, 4 mm for high power and 1.8 mm for the oil immersion.

4. The working media is air with low and high power objectives and cedar wood oil with oil immersion objective. The cedar wood oil has the same refractive index as the glass slide on which the object is placed.
5. The total working magnification of the compound microscope is equal to the eyepiece power X the objective power.

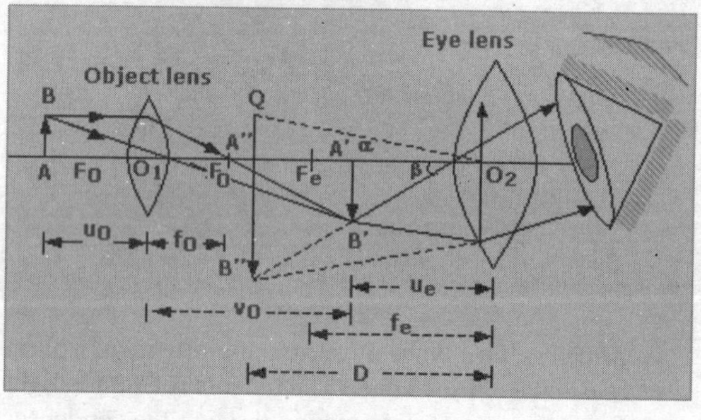

Fig. 1.2

As the magnification increases, the working length as well as the field size or area under observation decreases. The maximum resolution with a good optical microscope is 1 micron.

The low power objective is used to get an overall view of the object. The adjustments made while using the low power objective are:

1. Concave mirror is used.
2. Condenser is lowered.
3. Iris diaphragm is partially closed to decrease intensity of illumination.
4. Coarse adjustment screw is used to focus the image.
5. Magnification obtained is 100.

The high power objective is used to get a greater magnification (450) and to observe the object in greater detail. The adjustments made are:

1. Concave mirror is used.
2. Condenser is raised.
3. Iris diaphragm is partially opened to increase intensity of illumination.
4. First focus under low power and then turn to high power and use fine adjustment screw to focus the image.

Oil immersion objective is used to observe the object in still greater detail magnification (1000). The adjustments made are:

1. Plane mirror is used to get a parallel beam of light.
2. Condenser is fully raised.
3. Iris diaphragm is fully opened to get maximum intensity of illumination.
4. Cedar wood oil is used to avoid any distortion of image.

Maintenance of the Microscope

i. The microscope must be handled carefully.
ii. The eyepiece, objectives and the mirrors are to be cleaned with a clean dry cloth.
iii. The eyepiece and the objectives (particularly the oil immersion objective) after use should be cleaned with cotton soaked in xylene. The oil immersion objective should be cleaned with xylene every time after use (xylene removes the oil from the objective) and the other objectives periodically.

Source of Light

a. Natural day light; or
b. Artificial light–a bulb of 40 watts is most commonly used in the laboratories.

BLOOD SAMPLE

Blood: Blood is specialised tissue having a complex fluid in which several different types of cells are suspended. If

Table 1.1

Objective	*Working length*	*Numerical aperture*	*Magnification*	*Eyepiece magnification*	*Total magnification*
Low power	16 mm	0.30	10	10	100
High power	4 mm	0.60	45	10	450
Oil immersion	1.8 mm	1.30	100	10	1000

blood clotting is prevented by addition of anticoagulants, the cellular components can be spun down by centrifugation. The supernatant material is called *plasma,* containing proteins, organic and inorganic substances, hormones, antibodies etc.

Serum: If blood is permitted to clot, the fibrin mesh traps the cells and retracts. When this is centrifuged, the supernatant material is called the serum and is identical to plasma with the loss of fibrinogen and other clotting factors.

Methods of Collection of Blood

Important: Use your own sterile lancet/needle.

1. Finger Prick Method (Capillary Blood)

- Hands of the examiner and subject should be washed properly.
- Clean the tip of the ring or middle finger of the subject with a cotton swab dipped in spirit (for sterilization).
- Allow the fingertip to dry as spirit can cause haemolysis of blood and pain at the wound site.
- Using a sterile needle/lancet and without touching its cutting portion, hold it in the right hand between the thumb and three fingers and prick the finger deep enough to ensure a free flow of blood.
- Wipe the first drop of blood with a swab.
- Allow a drop of sufficient large size to form and take the sample.
- When adequate amount of blood has been obtained for the required experiment a sterile spirit swab is placed on the site of the prick with some pressure till the bleeding ceases.

Precautions

1. Do not squeeze the finger, as it will lead to the dilution of blood with tissue fluids, thereby giving low values and unreliable results.
2. The first drop of blood should be discarded as it contains damaged cells and fluid.

2. Collection of Venous Blood

- Use a sterile dry 10 ml syringe with a 21G needle.
- Rest the arm on the edge of the table. Identify a vein in the antecubital fossa. Clean the area with spirit and allow it to dry.
- Apply a tourniquet around the upper arm. Ask the subject to open and close the fist repeatedly so that the vein gets engorged.
- Introduce the needle under the skin and then puncture the vein from the side. When blood flows into the syringe, release the tourniquet and draw the required amount of blood.
- Withdraw the needle and apply a cotton swab over the site of puncture and apply pressure for 2 to 3 minutes till bleeding stops.
- Remove the needle from the syringe and expel collected blood into containers containing anticoagulants. Mix to prevent clotting.

3. Collection of Arterial Blood:

Blood can also be collected from an artery. This is done primarily for blood gas analysis (PO_2 and PCO_2).

ANTICOAGULANTS

These are substances used for preventing the clotting of blood and maintaining its fluidity. The most common agents are:

1. **Oxalates (of Ammonium or Potassium):** These act by precipitating calcium ions necessary for coagulation.
2. **Sodium Citrate (3.8%):** Action similar to oxalates.
3. **Heparin:** This is a natural anticoagulant present in circulation also available in synthetic form.
4. **EDTA (Ethylene Diamine Tetra Acetic Acid):** Acts as a calcium chelating agent.

DILUTING FLUIDS

For the estimation of various cellular components of blood, it is necessary to dilute the blood. The following diluting fluids are routinely used for various cell counts:

1. *Hayem's Fluid (for RBC count)*

Sodium chloride	:	0.5 gm
Mercuric chloride	:	0.25 gm
Sodium sulphate	:	2.5 gm
Distilled water to 100 ml		

2. *Turk's Fluid (for WBC count)*

Glacial acetic acid	:	3.0 ml
Gentian violet (1%)	:	1.0 ml
Distilled water to 100 ml		

3. *Reticulocyte Diluting Fluid*

Brilliant cresyl blue	:	1.0 gm
Sodium chloride	:	1.0 gm
Sodium citrate	:	3.8 gm
Distilled water to 100 ml		

4. *Rees-ecker Fluid (for platelet count)*

Sodium citrate	:	3.8 gm
Formaldehyde	:	0.2 ml
Brilliant cresyl blue	:	0.05 gm
Distilled water to 100 ml		

The solution is filtered and centrifuged at 7,500 rmp for 30 min and stored in refrigerator.

5. *Pilot's Solution (for eosinophil count)*

Pholoxine	:	1.0 gm
Propylene glycol	:	50.0 ml
Sodium carbonate (10%)	:	1.0 ml
Distilled water to 100 ml		

6. *Dunger's Solution (for eosinophil count)*

Aq. eosin 1%	:	5 ml
Acetone	:	5 ml
Sodium carbonate	:	1 ml
Distilled water to 100 ml		

STAINS

Leishman Stain (for DLC)

Leishman powder	:	0.15 gm (contains eosin and methylene blue)

Dissolved in acetone-free methyl alcohol and the volume made to 100 ml.

AIM

- **Handling the microscope and observation of the peripheral smears under various objectives of the microscope low power, high power and oil immersion. Note the difference and draw your observations.**
- **Observe and try to differentiate the various blood cells.**
  - Red blood cells
  - White blood cells
    Neutrophils
  - Eosinophils
  - Basophils
  - Lymphocytes
  - Monocytes
  - Platelets

2

HAEMOCYTOMETRY

AIM

1. To study the haemocytometer and to identify the squares used for RBC and WBC count on the improved Neubauer's counting chamber.
2. To practice dilution of the blood.
3. To charge the Neubauer's chamber for determining RBC and WBC counts.

MATERIALS

1. Microscope.
2. Haemocytometer (diluting pipettes and counting chamber).
3. Diluting fluids.
4. Materials for capillary puncture.

Description of the Apparatus

The Thoma-Zeiss haemocytometer consists of a Thomas RBC pipette, a Thomas WBC pipette and a ruled glass slide which is the counting chamber used for counting of blood cells called the improved Neubauer's chamber.

Pipettes

The pipettes are used to dilute the blood to a known dilution. Each has a narrow stem divided into 10 equal parts. The stem widens into a bulb with a bead in it. The bulb serves as a mixing chamber. The capacity of the bulb with respect to the stem varies for RBC and WBC pipettes. The bulb narrows above and to this end is attached a rubber tubing which ends in a mouthpiece.

The bead serves:

- In identification of the pipette;
- As a mechanical stirrer;
- To see if the pipette is dry or wet.

The following are the differences between RBC and WBC pipettes:

	RBC pipette	*WBC pipette*
1. Markings		
a. On the stem	0.5 and 1	0.5 and 1
b. Above the bulb	101	11
2. Capacity of the bulb	100 parts	10 parts
3. Bead	Red bead	White bead

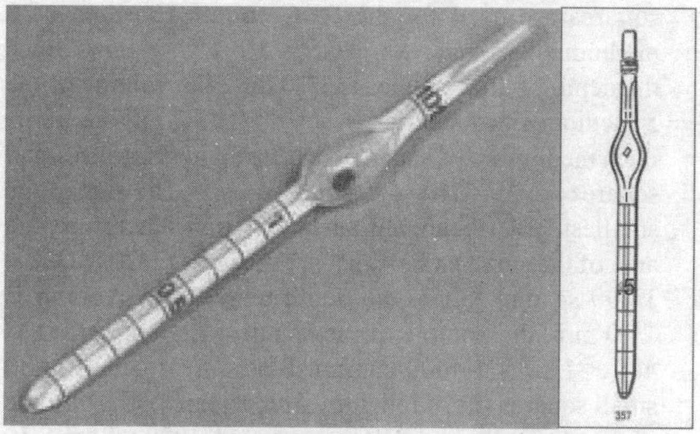

RBC pipette WBC pipette

Fig. 2.1

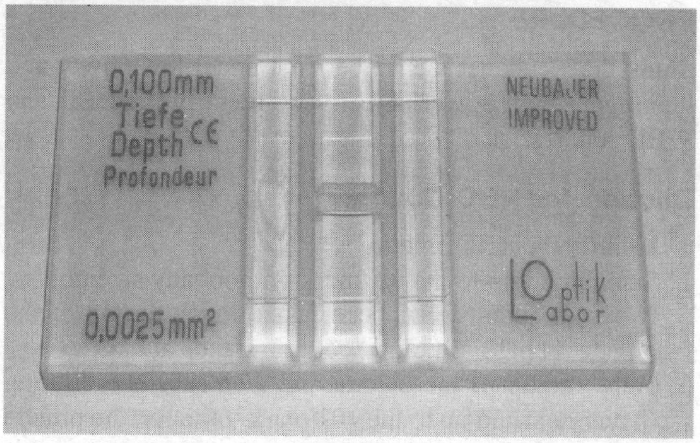

Fig. 2.2

Improved Neubauer's Counting Chamber

- This consists of a thick glass slide divided into two central platforms by an H-shaped groove.
- The central platform is slightly lower than the sides. When a cover slip is placed covering the central platform and resting on the side platforms, the depth under the cover slip and the central platform is 1/10 mm. When the chamber is charged with a drop of diluted blood, a thin film of fluid of known volume is got on the central platform and this is used for doing the cell counts.

- On the central platforms are engraved ruled squares used for various cell counts. The ruled area is a square measuring 3 mm × 3 mm. This area is divided into 9 large equal squares, each having an area of 1 sq. mm (1mm × 1mm). The four large corner squares are used for the WBC count while the large 1mm square in the center is used for the RBC count.
- Each of the WBC squares is further divided into 16 smaller squares each measuring 1/16 sq. mm.
- The 1 sq. mm central square for RBC is divided into 25 medium sized squares by means of triple lines. Each medium sized square measures 1/5 mm in length and has an area of 1/5 × 1/5 =1/25 sq. mm. The four-corner medium sized squares and the central medium sized squares are used for the RBC count. The area of 5 medium sized squares is 1/25 × 5 = 1/5 sq. mm. Since the depth of the chamber is 1/10 mm, the volume of the 5 medium sized squares is 1/5 × 1/10 = 1/50 cu. mm.
- Each medium sized square is further divided into 16 small squares i.e. 25 × 16 = 400 small squares. The side of the smallest RBC square measures 1/20 mm. Therefore, the area of the smallest RBC square measures 1/20 × 1/20 = 1/400 sq mm. Since the depth under the coverslip is 1/10 mm, the volume of the smallest RBC square is 1/400 × 1/10 = 1/4000 cu.mm. RBCs are counted in 80 small squares (i.e. 5 medium sized squares); the volume of the 80 small sized RBC squares is 1/4000 × 80 = 1/50 cu.mm.

PROCEDURE

Study the Neubauer's chamber first under low power and then under high power objectives. Identify the RBC and WBC squares.

Dilution for RBC Counts

1. Identify the RBC pipette.
2. Suck blood up to the 0.5 mark without any air bubbles. If excess quantity has been taken, touch the tip of the pipette on palm till blood column stands at 0.5.
3. Wipe the tip of the pipette and then suck the diluting (hayem's) fluid up to the 101 mark. Initially, the pipette is placed in the diluting fluid at an acute angle and it is gradually made vertical as it reaches the 101 mark.
4. Knot the rubber tubing of the pipette. Mix the contents by carefully rotating the pipette between the palm of your hand.
5. 0.5 part of blood is diluted to 100 parts, which is the capacity of the bulb to give a dilution of 1 in 200, hence fluid in stem of the pipette does not take part in dilution and is rejected before charging the chamber.

Dilution of WBC Count

1. Identify the WBC pipette.
2. Take the blood up to 0.5 mark. Wipe the tip and suck the WBC (Turk's) fluid up to the 11 mark to give a dilution of 1 in 20.

Charging the Neubauer's Chamber

1. Clean and dry the counting chamber and coverslip.
2. Place the counting chamber on the microscope stage.
3. Place the coverslip over the central platform.
4. Focus the chamber first under low power and identify the WBC and RBC squares. WBC is counted in low power and counts for RBC are done under high power.
5. Mix the contents of the blood prior to charging.
6. Discard the first two drops of fluid as the stem of the pipette contains only the diluting fluid.
7. Place the tip of the pipette on the central platform near the edge of the coverslip and allow a small amount of fluid to flow under the cover slip by capillary action taking care to avoid air bubbles and overflow into the troughs.
8. Allow the cells to settle for 1-2 minutes and study the cells and squares under the microscope after charging.
9. Take care to keep the Neubauer's chamber horizontal while studying the cells.
10. While counting consider all cells lying inside the square as well as all the cells lying only on the upper and left-hand boundary of the square. Discard cells on the lower and right hand boundary so as to avoid counting the cells twice.

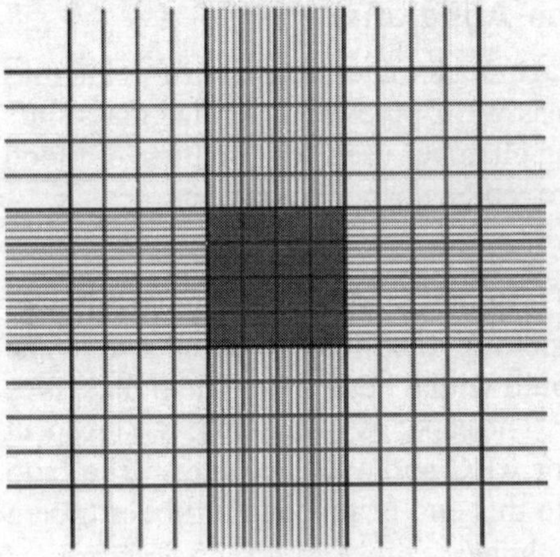

Fig. 2.3

Questions:

1. Draw a labelled diagram of the improved Neubauer's chamber.
2. Calculate the area and volume of fluid in the (i) Smallest RBC square (ii) Medium sized RBC square (iii) Large RBC square (iv) Large WBC square.
3. What is the need for having the '1' mark on the stem?
4. What other cell counts can the Neubauer's chamber be used for?

3

ESTIMATION OF HAEMOGLOBIN

AIM

To estimate the haemoglobin (Hb) concentration of blood by Sahli's method.

PRINCIPLE

This method is based on the haemolysis of RBCs from a known volume of blood and conversion of the Hb to acid haematin (dark brown in colour) by N/10 HCl. Haemoglobin is then estimated by dilution of the acid haematin formed with distilled water and its colorimetric matching with a suitable standard.

MATERIALS

1. Sahli's haemoglobinometer.
2. N/10 HCl.
3. Distilled water.
4. Materials for capillary puncture.

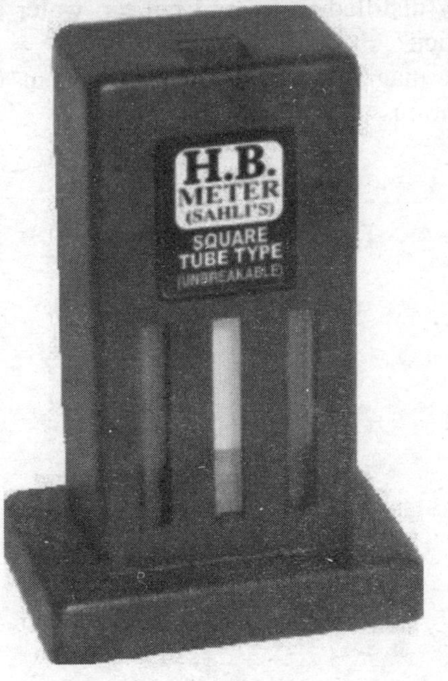

Fig. 3.1

Description of the Apparatus

- The haemoglobinometer is a rectangular box consisting of a groove to accommodate the 'haemoglobinometer tube'.
- The haemoglobinometer tube (which can be either round or square shaped) is graduated in percentage and/or in gm/100 ml. The tube can be taken out when required.
- The box also has a 'comparator' (brown stripes of glass representing coloured standards).
- The haemoglobin pipette has a single mark on it for measuring 0.02 ml (20 cu.mm) of blood.
- A glass stirrer is provided for mixing.

PROCEDURE

- With the help of a dropper take N/10 HCl up to the lowest mark (10% or 2 gm%) of the Hb tube.
- Taking aseptic precautions prick the fingertip. Discard the first drop of blood. From the next drop formed draw blood into the haemoglobin pipette up to the mark. 20 cu. mm taking care that there are no air bubbles in the column of blood drawn. If excess quantity of blood has been drawn touch the tip of the pipette on palm of the hand till the blood column stands at 20 cu. mm. Wipe the excess blood from the tip of the pipette.
- Transfer the blood immediately to the graduated Hb tube containing the N/10 HCl. Rinse the pipette twice or thrice by drawing the solution and expelling it back into the Hb tube (avoid frothing).
- Allow the solution to stand for 10 minutes, for the maximum conversion of Hb in blood sample to acid haematin, giving the solution a clear brown colour.
- Add distilled water drop by drop. Stir the contents well with the stirrer after each addition and match the colour of the solution with that of the standard on the comparator.
- Matching should be done against natural source of light when the plane surface of the tube is facing you and after lifting the stirrer out of the solution (but not out of the tube till final matching is done).

- Carry out the dilution till the colour of the mixture matches the colour of the standard plates in the comparator.
- When the colour matches with that of the standard take the reading of the lower meniscus on the graduated tube in gms of Hb per 100 ml of blood (gm%).
- Now add one drop of distilled water and match the colour once again. If it appears lighter take the previous reading but if it appears perfectly match repeat the above step.
- In this method on the percentage scale of Hb tube 100% =14.5gm of Hb/100ml of blood. It is a clinical representation and different instruments have different values for 100 % Hb. Therefore Hb reading on the gm% scale is preferred.

Precautions

1. Aseptic puncture should be made on ring finger of left hand. Commonly the ring finger is chosen as in case infection occurs it cannot spread to other areas of hand as its synovial sheath is not continuous with the palmer spaces like that of the other fingers. Moreover finger pulp or tip is rich in capillary network puncture is made there.
2. Accurate amount of acid and blood should be taken in the tube.
3. Rinse the pipette 2-3 times by drawing and expelling back the solution.
4. Distilled water to be added drop by drop and stirred every time.
5. Colour is matched when the stirrer is out of the solution but not completely out of the tube.

Other Methods

1. *Photoelectric colorimetric method:* It makes use of photoelectric colorimeter that measures the amount of light absorbed by a solution. Hb converted into:
   a. Cyanmethaemoglobin–By Drabkins reagent ($NaHCO_3$, potassium cyanide, potassium ferricyanide).
   b. Alkaline hematin–By addition of N/10 NaOH.
   c. Oxyhaemoglobin–By addition of ammonia.
2. *Haldane's method:* Haemolysis of RBCs in distilled water and addition of carbon monoxide, match colour with that of standard.
3. *Talliquist's method:* Matching the colour of a blood drop on a filter paper with that of a printed paper scale.
4. *Indirect method:* O_2 carrying capacity and iron content of the blood can be determined. 1gm% Hb when fully saturated combines with 1.34 ml O_2 therefore Hb concentration an index of oxygen carrying capacity of blood. In 1gm of Hb the iron content is 3.34 mg.

Questions:

1. What are your observations and give the normal range of values for haemoglobin?
2. What is the clinical importance of this experiment?
3. Name the common conditions in which Hb is high or low.
4. Calculate the oxygen carrying capacity of your blood.
5. How does Hb A differ from Hb F?
6. Discuss the advantages and disadvantages of Sahli's method.
7. Can N/10 HCl be used instead of distilled water for dilution and why?
8. Why concentrated acid cannot be used in this method?
9. Why haemoglobin has to be converted to another compound for colour estimation?
10. Why N/10 HCl is taken upto 2 gm% mark? What will happen to readings, if N/10 HCl is taken higher or lower than 2 gm% mark?
11. Why distilled water and not tap water are used for dilution?
12. Draw diagrams of the various components of the Sahli's apparatus.

4

RBC COUNT (RBC)

AIM

To determine the RBC counts in a unit of blood, i.e., per cu. mm. of blood.

PRINCIPLE

A measured quantity of blood is mixed with a diluting fluid, which is isotonic with blood. Dilution is necessary because in the normal blood the individual cells can hardly be distinguished in a counting chamber. A drop of this diluted fluid is placed in a counting chamber and the number of RBC's in a known volume is determined. The number of cells present in 1 cu. mm of undiluted blood can be determined by multiplying the number of cells in diluted by the dilution factor.

MATERIALS

1. Microscope.
2. Haemocytometer–Neubauer's chamber and RBC pipette.
3. RBC diluting fluid (Hayem's fluid).
4. Materials for capillary puncture.

DILUTING FLUID

It is known as Hayem's fluid and contains:
NaCl: 0.5 gm (maintains isotonicity).
$HgCl_2$: 0.25 gm (acts as a preservative, prevents formation of moulds, fungi).
Na_2SO_4: 2.5 gm (prevents rouleaux formation)
Distilled water to make 100 ml.

RBC PIPETTE

It is known as Thoma's red cell pipette. It consists of a stem and a bulb or mixing chamber. The stem is a graduated capillary tube. It has two marks on it: 0.5 and 1 mark. The stem is divided into 10 equal divisions. The stem opens into the bulb which has a red bead. The capacity of the bulb is 100 times more than the stem. The next mark is 101. The pipette is attached to a rubber tubing. The bead serves in identification of the pipette, serves as a mechanical stirrer and to know if the pipette is dry or not.

PROCEDURE

1. To collect the blood sample under aseptic precautions and to fill the pipette:

- Take RBC diluting fluid in a watch glass.
- Taking all aseptic precautions prick the finger, discard the first drop of blood and using a dry pipette, dip the pipette tip well in the second blood drop formed.
- Suck until the blood column reaches the mark 0.5 exactly. If excess quantity has been taken touch the tip of the pipette on palm till the blood column stands at 0.5. There should not be any air bubble in the column.
- Wipe off the excess blood from the tip of the pipette, dip well into the diluting fluid and suck the fluid till mark 101 is reached.
- Knot the rubber tube on pipette. Mix the contents by holding the pipette horizontally and carefully rotating the pipette on the palms of your hands.
- Having mixed the contents well the dilution of blood obtained is 1:200.

2. To charge the counting chamber:

- Clean and dry the counting chamber and coverslip.
- Place the counting chamber on the microscope stage.
- Put the coverslip across the side platforms so that it covers the Neubauer's ruling on the middle platform.
- Focus the field under low power.
- Discard the first two drops from the pipette because the stem of the pipette contains only diluting fluid.
- Place the next drop on the middle platform just near the margin of the coverslip. The tip should make 45° with coverslip.
- The drop instantly flows under the coverslip by capillary action.
- An ideally charged chamber is one, which has been charged with a single adequate sized drop, which just fills the chamber without leaving any air bubbles.

- If the fluid overflows into the gutters, it is called over-charging. If it is insufficient to fill the chamber or having air bubbles, it is said to be under-charged.
- Should the chamber be over or under-charged, the procedure is repeated after thoroughly cleaning the chamber and the coverslip with soap and water.
- The chamber should not be charged in parts by two or more smaller drops.
- Let the cells settle for1-2 minutes.

3. To count the red blood cells:

- Under high power of microscope the RBC looks like reddish brown discs, distributed all over the field.
- Identify and check the distribution of RBC's in the four corners and one central RBC squares. Recharge the chamber if distribution is not uniform.
- Count the total number of RBCs in the four corner squares and one central most square of the central square and enter results in squares provided.
- While counting, consider the cells lying on the upper and left hand boundary to be inside the square and those lying on the right and lower boundary outside.

Calculation

- Central square volume = 1mm × 1mm × 1/10 mm.
- Central square divided into 5 small squares. Therefore dimensions of each small square will be 1/5 × 1/5 × 1/10.
- Total number of cells in four corners and 1 central small squares of central RBC squares = n.
- n no. of RBCs in 5 small squares.
- Or n no. of RBCs present in 1/5 × 1/5 × 1/10 × 5 cu.mm.
- Or n no. of RBCs present in 1/ 50 cmm.
- Therefore in 1 cmm – 50 × n no. of RBCs present.
- Dilution is 1 in 200. Therefore RBC count/cmm in undiluted blood will be 50 n × 200/cu. mm i.e. 10,000 n/cu.mm.

Precautions

1. Prick should be aseptic and bold enough to give free flowing blood. At no stage finger should be squeezed to take out the blood.
2. Both haemocytometer and coverslip must be dry and free of grease.
3. Use only dry pipette (bead in the bulb should move freely).
4. Fill the pipette accurately with blood and diluting fluid.
5. Never use a broken coverslip.
6. Before charging the chamber the fluid in the stem of the pipette has to be discarded.
7. The coverslip should be placed symmetrically so as to cover the ruled area completely.
8. There should be no under or overcharging of the chamber (count will be low in both cases).
9. After charging the chamber allow 1-2 minutes for the cells to settle down but the count should be made before the fluid in the chamber starts drying up.
10. While counting the cells the stage of the microscope should not be tilted.

Questions:

1. What are your observations?
2. What is the normal RBC count?
3. What is the clinical importance of this experiment? What are the conditions in which RBC count increases or decreases?
4. Why a dilution of 200 times is needed in the case of total RBC count?
5. What are the other uses of the RBC pipette and the Neubauer's chamber?
6. What are the various sources of error in this experiment?
7. Does the presence of WBCs in the counting chamber affect the RBC count?

5 BLOOD INDICES (HAEMOGRAM)

After determining the values of RBCs, Hb and PCV, we can calculate various hematological indices, which are as follows:

Mean Corpuscular Volume: It is the average volume of a red blood cell in cubic microns.

$$\text{MCV} = \frac{\text{Volume of packed red cells in ml/liter of blood}}{\text{Red cells in millions/cu mm of blood}}$$

Normal value = $86 \pm 10\ \mu m^3$

Significance:

RBC's with normal MCV are k/a – NORMOCYTES

Increased MCV – MACROCYTES

Decreased MCV– MICROCYTES

Mean Corpuscular Haemoglobin: Average amount of haemoglobin in an erythrocyte expressed in picograms (pg). Amount of hemoglobin in picograms in a single red cell.

$$\text{MCH} = \frac{\text{Hb in gms/100 ml of blood}}{\text{RBC count in millions/cu mm of blood}} \times 100$$

Normal Value = 29.5 ± 2.5 pg

Mean Corpuscular Hemoglobin Concentration: It is the amount of hemoglobin per unit volume of red cell mass expressed as percentage.

MCHC is hemoglobin concentration in a single red cell or amount of Hb expressed as percentage of the volume of RBC.

$$\text{MCHC} = \frac{\text{Hb in gms/100 ml of blood}}{\text{Volume of packed cells/100 ml of blood}} \times 100$$

Normal range = 32-38%

Significance: If MCHC is within normal range → RBC's are k/a NORMOCHROMIC.

If MCHC is decreased→RBC's are known as HYPOCHROMIC.

COLOUR INDEX

$$\text{CI} = \frac{\text{Hb expressed as \% of normal}}{\text{RBC count expressed as \% of normal}}$$

Normal range=1 ± 0.15

Questions:

1. What is the importance of determining the values of blood indices or knowing haemogram?
2. Tabulate the various changes in the blood indices in the different types of anemia.
3. Why MCHC cannot be greater than the normal value?

6

TOTAL LEUCOCYTE COUNT (WBC)

AIM

To determine the number of leucocytes in one cu.mm of blood.

PRINCIPLE

A known volume of blood is diluted with a known volume of the diluting fluid and the number of WBCs in one cu.mm of diluted blood is determined. By knowing the dilution, the number of cells in one cu.mm of undiluted blood is calculated by multiplying the number of cells by the dilution factor.

MATERIALS

1. Microscope.
2. Hemocytometer (Neubauer's counting chamber and WBC pipette.
3. WBC diluting fluid (Turk's fluid).
4. Materials for capillary puncture.

DILUTING FLUID

It is known as Turk's fluid and it consists of:

Glacial acetic acid: 3 ml
Gentian violet 1%: 1 ml
Distilled water to make 100 ml

- Glacial acetic acid:
  - Destroys the RBCs.
  - Acts as a fixative.
  - Imparts refractility to cells.
- Gentian violet stains the nuclei of the WBCs.

WBC PIPETTE

This bears a stem and bulb. The bulb serves as a mixing chamber. The stem bears a 0.5 mark and a 1 mark. The bulb is 10 times the volume of the stem. There is also an 11 mark above the bulb. A white bead is present in the bulb. The bulb is connected to a rubber tube. The white bead serves in identification of the pipette for white blood cell and serves as a mechanical stirrer and to know if the pipette is dry or not.

PROCEDURE

1. **To collect the blood sample under aseptic precautions and to fill the pipette:**
   - Take WBC diluting fluid in a watch glass.
   - Taking all aseptic precautions prick the finger, discard the first drop of blood and using a dry pipette, dip the pipette tip well in the second blood drop formed.
   - Suck until the blood column reaches the mark 0.5 exactly. If excess quantity has been taken touch the tip of the pipette on palm till the blood column stands at 0.5. There should not be any air bubble in the column.
   - Wipe off the excess blood from the tip of the pipette, dip well into the diluting fluid and suck the fluid till mark 11 is reached.
   - Knot the rubber tube on pipette. Mix the contents by holding the pipette horizontally and carefully rotating the pipette on the palms of your hands.
   - Having mixed the contents well the dilution of blood obtained is 1:20.
2. **To charge the counting chamber:**
   - Clean and dry the counting chamber and coverslip.
   - Place the counting chamber on the microscope stage.
   - Put the coverslip across the side platforms so that it covers the Neubauer's ruling on the middle platform.
   - Focus the field under low power. The condenser of the microscope should be lowered.
   - Discard the first drop from the pipette because the stem of the pipette contains only diluting fluid.
   - Place the next drop on the middle platform just near the margin of the coverslip.
   - The drop instantly flows under the coverslip by capillary action.
   - An ideally charged chamber is one, which has been charged with a single adequate sized drop, which just fills the chamber without leaving any air bubbles.
   - If the fluid overflows into the gutters, it is called over-charging. If it is insufficient to fill the chamber or having air bubbles, it is said to be under-charged.

- Should the chamber be over or under-charged, the procedure is repeated after thoroughly cleaning the chamber and the coverslip with soap and water.
- The chamber should not be charged in parts by two or more smaller drops.
- Let the cells settle for 1-2 minutes.

3. To count the white blood cells:

- Under low power of microscope the WBCs looks like black dots, distributed all over the field. If in doubt the black dots can be observed under high power WBC will show as stained nuclei surrounded by colourless cytoplasm and the cell membrane. All other black dots are artifacts.
- Identify and check the distribution of WBC in the four corner WBC squares. Recharge the chamber if distribution is not uniform.
- Count the total number of WBCs in the four large corner squares and enter results in squares provided.
- While counting, consider the cells lying on the upper and left hand boundary to be inside the square and those lying on the right and lower boundary outside.

Calculations

- Area of each WBC square: 1 × 1=1 sq. mm.
- Area of 4 WBC squares: 4 sq. mm.
- Depth of the chamber: 1/10 mm.
- Volume of 4 squares: 4 × 1/10 =0.4 or 4/10 cu.mm.
- Total no. of cells in 0.4 cu.mm of diluted blood = n.
- Total no. of cells in 1 cu. mm of diluted blood = n/0.4.
- Dilution is 20 times, the total no. of cells in 1 cu mm of undiluted blood

  = (n × 20) / 0.4.

  = n × 50/cu mm.

Precautions

1. Prick should be aseptic and bold enough to give free flowing blood. At no stage finger should be squeezed to take out the blood.
2. Both haemocytometer and coverslip must be dry and free of grease.
3. Use only dry pipette (bead in the bulb should move freely).
4. Fill the pipette accurately with blood and diluting fluid.
5. Never use a broken coverslip.
6. Before charging the chamber the fluid in the stem of the pipette has to be discarded.
7. The coverslip should be placed symmetrically so as to cover the ruled area completely.
8. There should be no under or overcharging of the chamber (count will be low in both cases).
9. After charging the chamber allow 1-2 minutes for the cells to settle down but the count should be made before the fluid in the chamber starts drying up.
10. While counting the cells the stage of the microscope should not be tilted.

Questions:

1. What are your observations?
2. Give the normal range of TLC.
3. What is the clinical significance of this experiment?
4. List the physiological and pathological variations in the number of WBCs.
5. Define leucocytosis, leucopenia and leukemia.
6. What are the various sources of errors in this experiment?

7 PREPARATION AND STAINING OF A BLOOD SMEAR, IDENTIFICATION OF LEUCOCYTES AND DIFFERENTIAL LEUCOCYTE COUNT

AIM

To prepare and stain a blood smear to identify the different leucocytes in the smear and to do a differential leucocyte count (DLC).

MATERIALS

1. Materials for capillary puncture.
2. Glass slides.
3. Leishman stain.
4. Distilled water.
5. Cedar wood oil.
6. Microscope.

COMPOSITION OF LEISHMAN STAIN

Leishman stain consists of:

- Methylene blue (basic stain).
- Eosin (acidic stain).
- Acetone-free methyl alcohol (acts as a fixative, it should be acetone-free since the presence of acetone causes changes in the shape and size of cells and may produce lysis of cells).

PROCEDURE

Preparation of a Blood Smear

- Three glass slides are thoroughly cleaned with soap and water and dried. They are then passed over a flame to make them grease free.
- Taking all aseptic precautions a capillary puncture is made as in earlier experiments. The first drop of blood is wiped off.
- A moderate sized drop each is then taken on all the three microslides, towards one end of the slide. Take slide to the finger and not the finger to the slide.
- Another glass slide (spreader) with a smooth edge is held firmly between the thumb and the index finger of the right hand and is placed slightly in front of the blood drop at an angle of 45°.
- The blood is gently spread throughout the width of the spreader.
- With a swift forward movement of the spreader the blood is spread over the glass slide, taking care that the blood smear is trailing behind the spreader.
- It is then dried in air.

STAINING THE SMEAR

- Place the slides horizontally across two glass rods on a sink or staining tray.
- Put 8-12 drops of Leishman stain on the slide so as to cover the smear.
- After about 1-2 minutes (fixation time), double amount of distilled water is added and is mixed well with the stain by blowing air gently on the slide with the help of a dropper.
- If the dilution of the stain is correct, the fluid will have a greenish scum floating on the surface.
- The three smears are washed after 8 minutes (first slide), 9 minutes (second slide) and 10 minutes (third slide). This is the usual time taken for the cells to stain (staining time) but it may vary with different Leishman stains.
- The smears are washed under the running water by allowing the water to fall first on the thumb and then run from one end of the smear to the other. The smear should be washed until it acquires a pinkish tinge.
- After wiping the back of the slide, it is set upright to dry.
- The smear can then be seen first under low power objective. Then under high power and finally under the oil immersion objective of the microscope by putting a drop of cedar wood oil on the slide and allowing the lower end of the oil immersion lens of the microscope to dip in the drop of oil and adjusting the fine adjustment.

(For using the oil immersion objective, the condenser of the microscope should be at highest position, the iris diaphragm should be fully open and the plain mirror should be used).

- Identification of cells and differential count should be done under oil immersion objective.
- Cells lying on the extreme end of the smear should not be counted.

Criteria of a Good Blood Smear

1. It should cover almost 2/3rd of the width and length of the slide.
2. It is tongue shaped with a head, body and tail end.
3. It is neither too thin nor too thick (a thick smear when placed on a white background appears red).
4. There are no longitudinal/cross striations or air gaps in the smear, or irregular long tails.

IDENTIFICATION OF DIFFERENT LEUCOCYTES

A stained blood smear would show:

1. *Red blood cells:* It is the most abundant cell type found anywhere in the smear. They are seen as light pink, non-nucleated, biconcave discs of uniform size (7.2 μ) and shape.
2. *White blood cells:* These are nucleated cells of various types. While identifying the various types of WBCs keep the following factors in mind in the given order:
   (a) The size of cells (as compared to RBCs).
   (b) Staining characteristics of cytoplasm and granules.
   (c) Type of nucleus.

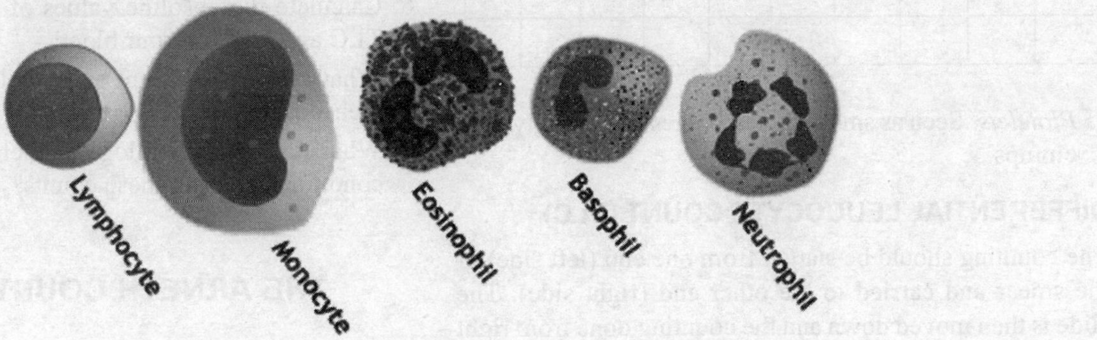

***MORPHOLOGICAL FEATURES OF VARIOUS LEUCOCYTES**

Leucocyte	*Cell size*	*Cytoplasm and granules*	*Nucleus*	N:C ratio	*%*
I. Granulocytes					
1. Neutrophil	10-14 μ	Plenty, pale pink in colour with fine pinkish violet granules	Multilobed, generally the lobes vary from 2-6 in number. Chromatin is coarse and ropy		50-70%
2. Eosinophil	10-14 μ	Pinkish in colour, contains coarse, brick red granules	Generally bilobed (spectacle shaped), stains bluish purple. Chromatin is coarse and ropy		1-4%
3. Basophils	10-14 μ	Light pink in colour with coarse blue granules, which almost obscure the nucleus	'S' shaped, purplish blue in colour with coarse chromatin		0-1%
II. Agranulocytes		**No granules seen with Leishman stain**		**N:C ratio**	
1. Lymphocyte	7-10 μ (small) 10-14 μ (large)	Scanty, pale blue in colour; forms a thin rim around the nucleus	Round or oval or indented and bluish purple in colour, occupies almost the whole of the cell. Chromatin is coarser and lumpy	About 80%	20-40%
2. Monocyte	14-18 μ	Plenty, bluish in colour	Oval or round or kidney shape, bluish-purple in colour, eccentric. Chromatin is finely reticular	About 50%	2-8%

N:C ratio = nucleus:cytoplasm ratio.

*. These features could also be seen in the above figures of each cell.

(d) The nuclear cytoplasmic ratio.
(For details refer to the following table).

OBSERVATION TABLE

3. *Platelets:* Seen as small stained bodies lying singly or in clumps.

DIFFERENTIAL LEUCOCYTE COUNT (DLC)

The counting should be started from one end (left side) of the smear and carried to the other end (right side). The slide is then moved down and the counting done from right to left. This procedure ensures that the same cells are not counted again and again. The extreme ends should not be counted, as the smear is likely to be too thick or too thin in these regions. The above procedure can be continued till a minimum of 100 cells has been counted. The type of leucocytes counted can be entered in the observation table provided by the first letter of the nomenclature of each type of WBC as N, L, M, E and B. Finally by counting each type of leucocyte marked on the paper, the percentage can be calculated.

PRECAUTIONS

1. The slides should be clean and grease-free; therefore, these should be cleaned thoroughly with soap and water immediately before use.
2. The glass spreader should be carefully selected. It should have a smooth and clean edge. If a rough-edged spreader is used, many of the leucocytes accumulate at the edges and in the tail of the smear. Also, a gross qualitative irregularity in distribution of cells will occur.
3. Make about 4-5 blood films so that at least one is satisfactory.
4. Mark the smeared surface with a glass marking pencil.
5. Do not heat dry or blot dry the smear.
6. Stored blood should not be used for making the smear.
7. The smear should be stained not later than 2 hours after it has been prepared.
8. Assess the quality of the smear, both grossly and microscopically (under low power) before staining it.
9. Only properly stained slide should be examined under the oil-immersion lens.

Questions:

1. Draw a diagram of all the WBCs seen in the smear.
2. Why should the stain be left undiluted initially for 1-2 minutes?
3. Why should the dilution be done with distilled water only? How does the pH influence the staining?
4. What is the function of cedar wood oil?
5. Discuss the significance of DLC.
6. Calculate the absolute values of various WBC's from TLC and DLC of your blood.
7. What are Arneth count and Schilling index? What are their different stages?
8. What are the physiological factors and pathological conditions altering these counts?

THE ARNETH COUNT or INDEX

AIM

To determine the percentage distribution of neutrophils on the basis of number of nuclear lobes.

THEORY

- The number of lobes in any neutrophil nucleus depends upon the cell's age, the older cells having large number. A neutrophil leucocyte showing unlobed, but deeply indented nucleus is a very young cell and one showing a five or six lobed nucleus indicates a stage prior to its final dissolution.
- According to the number of lobes of nucleus, the neutrophils are classified into five stages.

Classification and percentages of neutrophil leucocytes (Arneth Index)

Nucleus	*Stage*	*Normal percentage*	*Stage of maturity*
Unlobed (N1)	I	5%	Newly formed
2-lobed (N2)	II	30%	
3-lobed (N3)	III	45%	Fully mature and functionally most efficient
4-lobed (N4)	IV	18%	
5-lobed (N5)	V	2%	Senile

Clinical Significance

1. Shift to left (regenerative shift): Stage I + II + III >80% indicates hyperactive functioning of the bone marrow e.g. Pyogenic infection, haemorrhage.
2. Shift to right (degenerative shift): Stage IV + V >20% indicates hypoactive bone marrow e.g., Aplasia of bone marrow.

Materials

Glass slides, microscope, Leishman's stain.

Procedure

- Prepare and stain a blood smear with Leishman's stain focus under the oil immersion objective.
- Identify neutrophils and note the number of nuclear lobes in each neutrophil.
- Count at least 100 neutrophils and enter the findings in a big square which has been divided into 100 small squares.
- For counting the cells, start from one end of the smear and proceed in a zig-zag manner as shown in the experiment on DLC.
- According to the number of lobes of the nucleus, the neutrophils are designated as N1, N2, N3, N4 and N5.
- On this basis, the neutrophils are referred to as stage I, II, III, IV and V respectively. Determine the percentage of the various stages of neutrophils. Express your results as percentage.
- Plot a graph with your observed values with neutrophil types on the X axis and the number of cells on the Y axis.

Questions:

1. What is the clinical significance of doing count / Arneth Index?
2. What is meant by "shift to the left/right" with respect to Arneth count? Give examples for each.
3 What is Arneth curve?

OBSERVATION TABLE

THE SCHILLING INDEX

- Schilling employed a similar classification of neutrophils, but included bone-marrow elements also.
- In this index, the following four stages are recognised:

Classification of neutophil leucocytes (Schilling Index)

	Nucleus	*Stage*	*Nomenclature*
1.	Single spherical nucleus	I	Myelocyte
2.	Slightly indented nucleus	II	Young metamyelocyte
3.	Lobulation seen in nucleus (corresponds to Arneth Stage I)	III	Older metamyelocyte (i.e. Band cell)
4.	2 to 5 lobed nucleus (Arneth stages 2 to 5)	IV	Older neutrophils

8

BLEEDING TIME (BT) AND CLOTTING TIME (CT)

BLEEDING TIME

AIM

To determine the bleeding time.

THEORY

Bleeding time is the time taken from the puncture of the blood vessel to the stoppage of bleeding.

It is a test of platelet function and integrity of capillary wall.

METHODS

1. Duke's Method.
2. Ivy's Method.

Duke's Method

Materials

- Materials for capillary puncture.
- Filter paper.
- Stop watch.

Procedure

- Set the stop watch at 'zero.'
- Under aseptic conditions a puncture is made to a depth of 2-3 mm on the fingertip, so that a free flow of blood results without squeezing.
- Stopwatch is started as soon as the puncture is made. Time of puncture of the finger is referred as **zero time**.
- The oozing blood is blotted gently with the filter paper after 30 seconds.
- Repeat the procedure in every 30 seconds using a fresh area on each occasion until bleeding stops and no further blood spot appears on the filter paper.
- Therefore each blot of blood on the filter paper represents 30 seconds flow of blood. The time is to be marked appropriately against each blood spot on the filter paper.
- Count the number of blood spots on the filter paper and multiply this by ½. This will give the BT in minutes.
- Normal bleeding time by this method is 2-6 minutes.

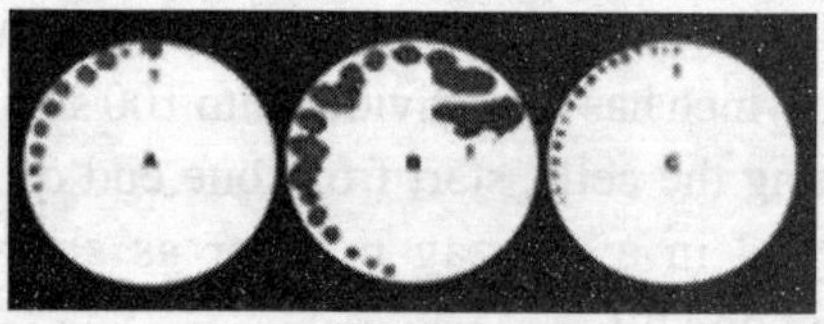

Fig. 8.1

Precautions

1. Finger should be pricked by a single stabbing action to give free flowing blood. At no stage should it be squeezed to obtain the blood.
2. Be alert and carefully note the 'zero time'.

IVY'S Method

Materials

- Sphygmomanometer.
- 70% ethanol or spirit.
- Sterilized lancet.
- Filter paper.
- Stopwatch.

Procedure

- A sphygmomanometer cuff is placed around the patient's upper arm and inflated to 40 mm of mercury, this is maintained through out the test.
- The volar surface of the forearm is cleaned with 70% ethanol and two separate punctures 5-10 cm apart are made in quick successions using the sterilized lancet and stopwatch is started. Care should be taken to avoid puncturing very superficial veins in people with thin skins.
- Blood exuding from each puncture is blotted completely on a filter paper at an interval of 15 seconds and the bleeding times of the two punctures are recorded separately and marked appropriately.

- The longer of the two bleeding times is probably a more accurate assessment of the result of the test than the average of the two.
- Normal value of bleeding time by this method is 1-9 minutes.

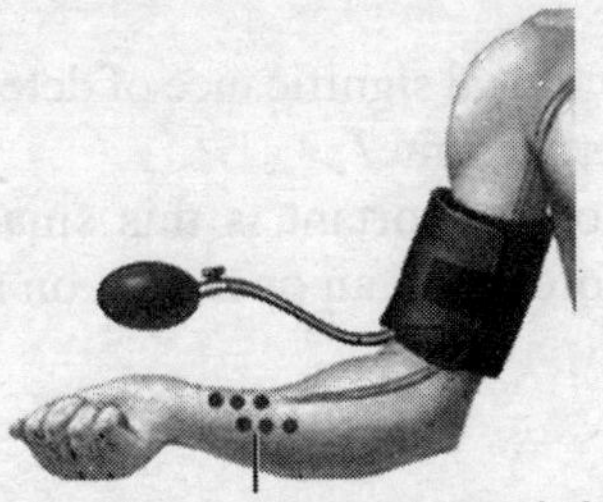

Two incisions are made and the time for stoppage of bleeding is recorded

Fig. 8.2

Questions:

1. What are the results of the experiment? Paste your results and analyse them.
2. Define bleeding time.
3. What are the factors on which bleeding time depends?
4. Name some conditions where the bleeding time is prolonged.
5. Explain the role of platelets in the arrest of bleeding.

CLOTTING TIME

AIM

To determine the clotting time.

THEORY

It is the time taken from the puncture of the blood vessel to the formation of a fibrin thread.

METHODS

1. Capillary glass tube method (Wright's method).
2. Lee and White Method.

Capillary Glass Tube Method

Materials

- Materials for capillary puncture.
- Capillary glass tubes of length 8-10 cm and bore diameter 1 mm.
- Stopwatch.

Procedure

- Under all aseptic conditions a capillary puncture is made on the fingertip sufficient enough to cause a free flow of blood.
- Stopwatch is started as soon as the puncture is made.
- The end of a glass capillary tube is introduced into the blood drop and blood enters the tube by capillary action.
- Hold the capillary tube filled with blood in the palm of the hand so as to maintain it close to body temperature.
- About 1 cm length of the tube is broken every 30 seconds till fibrin threads are seen in between the two broken tips and the time is noted.
- Arrange the broken pieces of the capillary tube, including the pieces with the fibrin thread in between the broken ends, on a filter paper. Mark the time below each piece. Preserve the pieces under a strip of cellotape. Paste this labelled paper in the file.
- The total time taken from the time of puncture (zero time) till the formation of a fibrin thread is the CT.
- Normal value of clotting time by this method is 2-6 minutes.

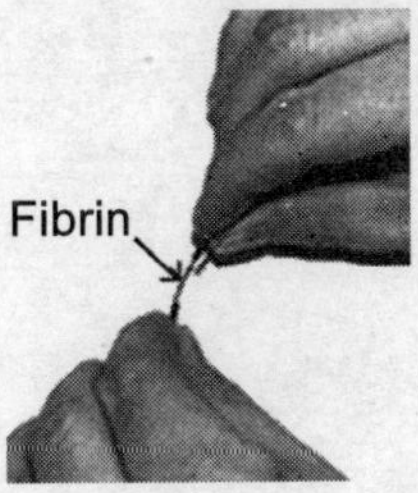

Fig. 8.3

Precautions

1. Glass capillary tube should never be filled with blood by means of sucking at the other end of the tube.
2. Strictly follow the procedure steps and preferably the experiment should be carried out at normal body temperature of 37°C.

Lee and White Method

Materials

- Materials for venepuncture.
- Four clean unsiliconized tubes of 10 mm bore.
- Water bath at 37°C.

Procedure

- Venous blood is withdrawn into a dry siliconized glass syringe and after detaching the needle, 1 ml volume is delivered into each of the four clean unsiliconized tubes, previously warmed to 37°C and kept in a water bath.
- A stopwatch is started as soon as the blood enters the syringe.
- The tubes are then gently tilted every minute, until one can be tilted through an angle greater than 90° without spilling the blood.
- The remaining tubes are then examined at half-minute intervals.
- The clotting time is taken as the average of the clotting time in the four tubes.

- Normal value of clotting time by this method in unsiliconized tubes is 8-18 minutes and in siliconized tubes is 20-60 minutes.

Questions:

1. What is your clotting time? Paste the labelled filter paper in the file.
2. Define clotting time. What are the factors on which clotting time depends?
3. Name the conditions where the clotting time is prolonged.
4. How does bleeding time differ from clotting time. Name a disease where both are altered.
5. How the clotting time is affected in siliconized and unsiliconized glass tubes?
6. What is the role of platelets in clotting and in clotting time?
7. What is the clinical significance of determining bleeding time and clotting time?
8. Visualise how important is this small exercise for a surgeon before doing an operation on a patient?

9 DETERMINATION OF BLOOD GROUPS (ABO & Rh)

AIM

To determine the blood group of your own blood.

PRINCIPLE

A suspension of red cells in citrated saline is treated with specific test sera and the presence or absence of agglutination is confirmed with the help of microscope. Basically it is based on antigen (in RBC) and antibody (in serum) reaction.

Materials

1. Citrated saline.
2. Anti-A and Anti-B sera.
3. Anti-D sera.
4. Materials for capillary puncture.
5. Glass/wooden stirrers.
6. Microscope.
7. Glass slides.
8. Dropper.

ABO GROUPING

Slide Method

- A suspension of red cells in citrated saline is prepared by adding a drop of blood to nine drops of citrated saline in a watch glass.
- Two clean glass slides are taken. A drop of anti-A serum is placed on the left half of the first slide and marked anti A while a drop of anti-B is put on the second slide and marked anti-B. A drop of saline is placed on the right half of these slides to serve as a control.
- A drop of red cell suspension is added to these drops and gently mixed with glass/wooden stirrer. Separate stirrers should be used for each test serum.
- The glass slides are gently rocked for about 3-5 min to effect a thorough admixture of red cell suspension with the test sera and saline.
- Observe the serum-cell mixtures for agglutination (clumping). Compare it with the cells in the saline control.
- Confirm your findings by observing the slides under the low power of a microscope.
- Record the presence or absence of agglutination in each slide and interpret the results as per the table given below.

Test Tube Method

Two small test tubes are taken and in each a drop of red cell suspension is taken. The test tube are labelled as anti-A and anti-B and corresponding serum is added to each and the contents are mixed well. The presence or absence of agglutination is confirmed under the microscope.

Blood Group	*Anti-A serum*	*Anti-B serum*	*Agglutinogen*	*Agglutinin*
A	+	—	A	β (anti-B)
B	—	+	B	α (anti-A)
AB	+	+	A & B	—
O	—	—	—	α (anti-A) β (anti-B)

+ : Agglutination – RBCs are massed together in clumps and lose their outline.

— : No agglutination – RBCs remain separated and evenly distributed.

Rh GROUPING

The procedure is same as above, except that anti-D serum is used in place of anti-A or anti-B serum. Observe for agglutination. Presence of agglutination is termed "Rh-positive" and absence of agglutination is termed as "Rh-negative".

The term "Rh-positive"(Rh+ve) as it is generally used means that the individual has agglutinogen D. The "Rh-negative" (Rh–ve) individual has no D antigen.

Observations

Anti-A serum	Anti-B serum	Anti-D serum
Blood group		

+ : Agglutination – : No agglutination

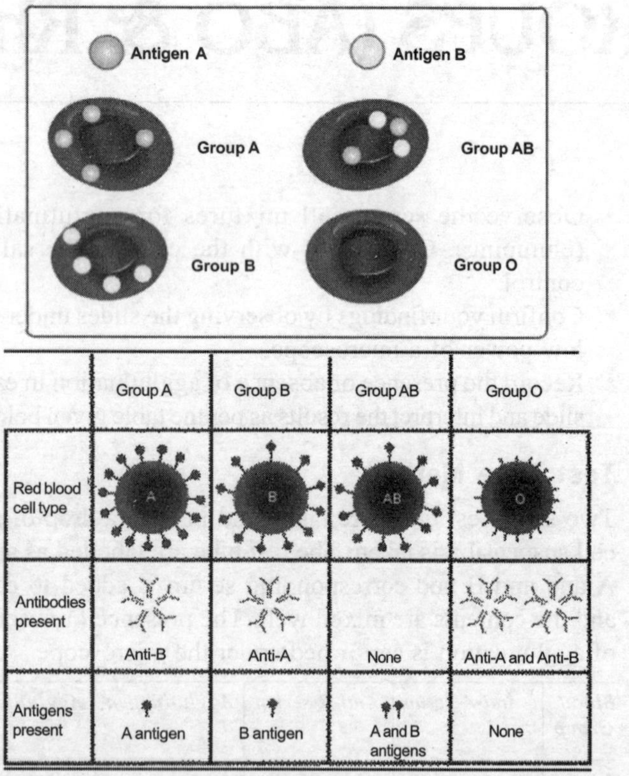

Fig. 9.1

Precautions

1. The slides should be thoroughly cleaned with soap and water.
2. The slides should be labelled before hand after placing the antisera A and B.
3. Separate stirrers should be used to prevent intermixing of the sera.
4. The slide should be examined for agglutination before solution dries up. Confirm the findings under low power of the microscope.
5. Undiluted blood should never be mixed with antisera directly, otherwise false positive results may develop.

Questions:

1. What is the importance of blood grouping?
2. What is the use of control in this experiment?
3. What could be the possible errors while doing this experiment?
4. What is the difference between coagulation, rouleaux formation and agglutination?
5. Which agglutinogens and agglutinins are present in your blood?
6. To whom can you donate blood and from whom can you accept blood?
7. What does anti-A and anti-B sera contain?
8. What is "cross matching" of blood?
9. What is Landsteiner's law? Discuss its applicability to various blood groups.
10. What are the various other blood groups and their importance?
11. What are the precautions you should take before blood transfusion?
12. Visualise how important is to know your blood group in day to day life where you may need blood transfusion or donate blood to others to save life.
13. Can the blood group be helpful in medicolegal cases of disputed paternity?

10

SPECIFIC GRAVITY OF BLOOD

AIM

To determine the specific gravity of the given sample of blood.

METHODS

1. **Direct Method:**
   In this, the weights of blood and the same volume of water are determined using capillary tubes called **pyenometers** and the ratio calculated.
2. **Indirect Method:**
   Principle: These are based on the law of floattation. A substance floats in a liquid if the density of the liquid is greater than that of the substance. The substance sinks in the liquid if the density of the liquid is less than that of the substance. If the densities of the substance and the liquid are equal, the substance gets suspended in the liquid.

1. HAMMER SCHLAG'S METHOD

Materials

- Benzene.
- Chloroform.
- Hydrometer.
- Sample of blood.

Procedure

- Benzene-chloroform mixture is prepared by adding 7.1 ml of benzene and 2.9 ml of chloroform. The mixture is taken in a glass cylinder.
- A drop of blood is added to the mixture from a height of 1 cm from the surface of the solution and its movement observed.
- Benzene is lighter than blood and chloroform is denser than blood. If the drop rises to the surface, benzene is slowly added to the mixture till the blood drop gets suspended in the mixture. If the drop sinks, chloroform is added slowly till the drop gets suspended.
- If the drop is suspended i.e. if it is stationary, the specific gravities of blood and the mixture are the same. The specific gravity of the mixture is then determined using a hydrometer.

2. PHILLIPS-VAN SLYKE METHOD

Materials

- Copper sulphate solutions (of specific gravity ranging between 1.050 to 1.064).
- Sample of blood.
- Test tubes.
- Dropper.

Procedure

- A graded series of copper sulphate solutions of specific gravity ranging between 1.050 and 1.064 is prepared and put into test tubes appropriately marked.
- A drop of blood is added from a height of 1 cm into each one of the solutions and the movement of the drop is noted.
- Due to the momentum, the blood drop first sinks to a depth of 2-3 cm below the surface of the solution but then it either rises to the surface, remains suspended or sinks down to the bottom depending on the specific gravity of blood sample.
- The specific gravities of the solutions wherein it gets suspended are noted.
- The blood drop remains discrete in the $CuSO_4$ solutions due to a covering of copper proteinate layer, which is stable for 15-20 seconds.

Normal specific gravity: Plasma : 1.026-1.031
RBC's : 1.092-1.095
Blood : 1.052-1.063

Questions:

1. Draw and note down your observations.

2. Define specific gravity.
3. Name the factors affecting the specific gravity of blood.
4. What are the physiological and pathological conditions that affect specific gravity of blood?
5. What is the clinical significance of determining specific gravity?
6. Why does the reading need to be taken immediately i.e. 15-20 seconds after the addition of the drop?

11

ERYTHROCYTE SEDIMENTATION RATE (ESR), PACKED CELL VOLUME (PCV) AND OSMOTIC FRAGILITY

ERYTHROCYTE SEDIMENTATION RATE (ESR)

AIM

To determine the ESR of blood.

ESR is the rate at which RBCs settle down when blood, to which an anticoagulant is added, is allowed to stand undisturbed in a narrow tube for one hour. The ESR is expressed in mm of clear plasma at the end of 1st hour.

Materials

- Westergren's tube and stand/rack.
- 3.8% sodium citrate.
- Vial.
- Dropper.

Description of Apparatus

Westergren Tube is 300 mm in length with an internal bore of 2.5 mm and is open at both the ends. It is a graduated pipette from 0 to 200 mm (only along the lower 2/3rd of its length). The tall rack for holding the pipette vertically is provided with rubber corks at the lower end and clips or screws at the upper end.

Procedure

- Using aseptic precaution draw 2 ml of venous blood from any convenient vein (anticubital vein is preferred) and gently mix it with 3.8% sodium citrate solution in a vial. The proportion of anticoagulant and blood is kept 1:4.
- Anticoagulated blood is sucked in the Westergren pipette uptill the '0' mark.
- Close the upper end immediately to prevent the blood from running out of the other end.
- Place it vertically on the Westergren stand by pressing the lower end of the pipette tightly on a rubber pad (vial cover) placed on the lower end of the stand and fixing it in place by screws provided on the upper end of the stand.
- Note the time and take the reading for ESR after the end of one hour.

Normal Values (Westergren's)

i. *Males:* 3-5 mm at the end of 1 hour.
ii. *Females:* 4-7 mm at the end of 1 hour.

Precautions

1. Arrange and check all the apparatus before starting the experiment.
2. Ensure all glass apparatus like tubes, pipette, dropper etc. are clear and absolutely dry.
3. Once the blood has been drawn after a venepuncture, detach the needle from the syringe and then gently transfer the blood into the bottle, otherwise haemolysis might occur.
4. Anticoagulant should be taken in the specific amount for a given method.
5. There should be no air bubble while filling the Westergren's or Wintrobe's tube with blood.
6. The tubes should be vertical.
7. While determining ESR note the time of fixing the pipette/tube and note the readings exactly after one hour.
8. Fill the pipette again in the event of escape of blood during fixing.

Questions:

1. What is the clinical significance of PCV?
2. Is there any difference between arterial and venous PCV?
3. Enumerate various factors which influence the process of sedimentation.
4. Why ESR reading is taken at the end of first hour?
5. Give the variations of ESR.
6. What is the clinical significance of ESR?

PACKED CELL VOLUME (PCV)

AIM

Packed Cell Volume (PCV) is the volume of cellular elements per unit volume of whole blood. It is expressed as a percentage or as ml per 100 ml of blood. It is composed of a lower column of red blood cells (VPRC) and an upper 'buffy' coat (layer) consisting of leucocytes and platelets.

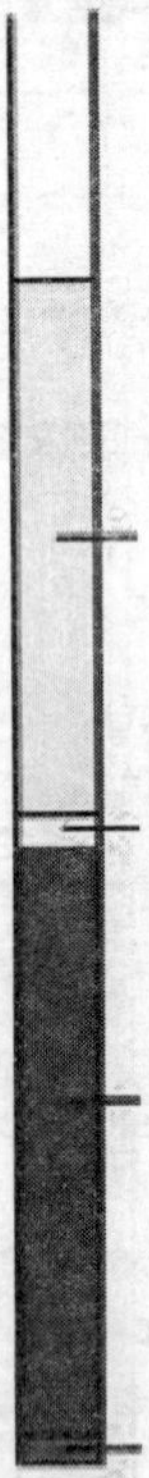

Fig. 11.1

Method

Wintrobe's method.

Materials

- Wintrobe's tube and stand/rack.
- Wintrobe's pipette.
- Venous blood.
- Anticoagulant double oxalate.
- Centrifuge machine.

Description of Apparatus

Wintrobe's Tube: It is 11 cm in length with an internal bore of 2.5 mm. It is calibrated in both directions from 0-10 and 10-0. Each cm has also been worked in millimeters. The markings 10-0 from above downwards are used for reading PCV (The markings 0-10 from downwards can be used for ESR estimation).

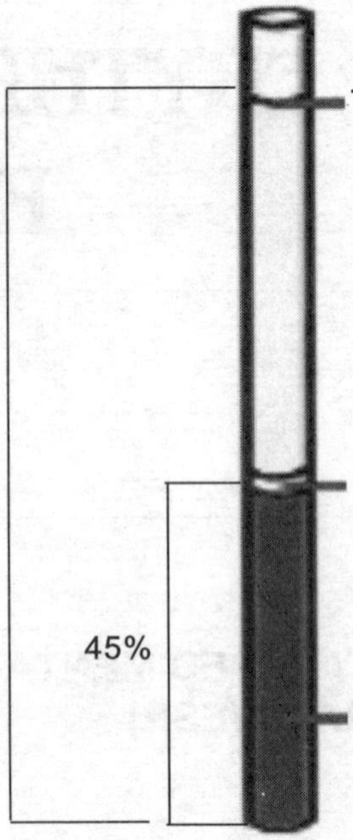

Fig. 11.2: Hematocrit tube

Procedure

- Using aseptic precaution draw 3 ml of venous blood from any convenient vein (anticubital vein is preferred) and gently mix it with a powdered mixture of double oxalate anticoagulant (a mixture of ammonium and potassium oxalate in the ratio of 3:2) in a vial.
- 2 ml of this blood is taken in the Wintrobe's pipette. The pipette is then introduced right down the bottom of the Wintrobe's tube and the blood is transferred into it slowly while gradually withdrawing the pipette out of the tube. The tube is filled upto the 10 mark on PCV side.
- No air bubble should be present in the tube.
- The tube is then centrifuged at the speed of 3000 revolutions/min. for 30 minutes.
- The tube is taken out and examined. The following columns (layers) can be seen from top to bottom:
  - Plasma layer.
  - Buffy coat (1 mm).
  - Column of RBCs.
- The height of the column of RBCs is read in mm and expressed as a %.

Normal Values

Adult man: Avg. 45% (Range-40 to 50%).
Adult woman: Avg. 42% (Range-37 to 47%).

EFFECTS OF HYPOTONIC, ISOTONIC AND HYPERTONIC SOLUTIONS ON RBCs

AIM

To show the effects of hypotonic, isotonic and hypertonic saline on RBCs.

Materials

- Saline solutions of 0.4%, 0.9% and 2.0% concentration.
- Glass slides.
- Microscope.
- Material for capillary puncture.

Procedure

- After taking the usual aseptic precautions a capillary puncture is made and a drop of blood is placed in the center of each of the three glass slides suitably marked.
- A few drops of hypotonic saline (0.4%), are added to first, isotonic (0.9%) to the second, and hypertonic saline (2.0%) to the third slide and the contents are thoroughly mixed in each case using separate thin sticks.
- After waiting for a few seconds a coverslip is placed on each of the glass slides and viewed under the high power objective of the microscope. The changes in size and shape of red cells in each of these solutions are noted.

Questions:

1. What are isotonic, hypertonic and hypotonic solutions?
2. What are the changes occurring when RBCs are placed in hypertonic, hypotonic and isotonic solutions? Why?
3. Draw diagrams of your observation.

OSMOTIC FRAGILITY TEST OF RED BLOOD CELLS

AIM

To determine the osmotic fragility of the given sample of blood.

Principle

The ease with which the red cells are broken down i.e. hemolysed in hypotonic solution is called osmotic fragility of red cells. It is determined by placing the cells in a graded series of hypotonic solutions and noting the concentrations of the solutions in which the cells are hemolysed.

Materials

- A graded series of NaCl solutions of concentrations ranging from 0.8% to 0.1%.
- Normal Saline (0.9%).
- Distilled water.
- Test tubes.
- Sample of blood.

Procedure

- A graded series of NaCl solutions of concentrations ranging from 0.8% to 0.1%, are taken in different test tubes placed in a rack.
- Test tubes containing normal saline (0.9%) and distilled water are also placed on either side of the graded saline solutions.
- A drop of blood is added, to each of the test tubes.
- The tube is then gently inverted once and allowed to stand for 30 min to allow the solution and distilled water to act on the RBCs.
- The test tubes are then centrifuged.
- If hemolysis occurs the solution in that test tube will be tinted red.
- The result is expressed in terms of the concentrations of NaCl in the two solutions in which are present the minimal and maximal detectable hemolysis respectively. Under normal conditions hemolysis starts when the concentration of the solution is 0.44% and is complete at 0.28%.

Questions:

1. What are your observations? Draw your findings.
2. What is the purpose of using the test tubes containing normal saline and distilled water.
3. What is hemolysis? What are its causes?
4. What is the normal osmotic fragility?
5. What happens to the fragility in?
   (a) Iron deficiency anemia
   (b) Sickle cell anemia
   (c) Hereditary spherocytosis. Why?
6. What are the factors which affect osmotic fragility?

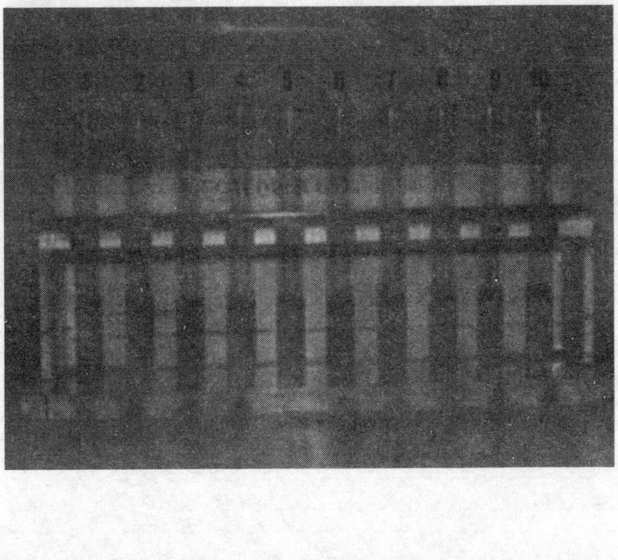

Fig. 11.3

12 PLATELET COUNT

AIM

To determine the number of platelets present per cubic mm of blood.

Method

Rees and Ecker method.

Materials

- RBC pipette.
- Hemocytometer.
- Microscope.
- Material for capillary puncture.
- Rees and Ecker fluid.

Composition of Rees and Ecker Fluid

- Sodium citrate – 3.8 gm (anticoagulant).
- Formaldehyde – 0.2 ml (fixative).
- Brilliant cresyl blue – 0.05 gm (stains platelets).
- Distilled water to make 100 ml.

The diluting fluid is filtered before use.

Procedure

- A capillary puncture is made on the fingertip, after taking the usual aseptic precautions. The first drop of blood is discarded.
- Blood is drawn into the RBC pipette upto 0.5 mark.
- The diluting fluid is drawn into the pipette till it reaches 101 mark. The blood and the diluting fluid are mixed thoroughly by rolling the pipette on the palm.
- After discarding a few drops from the pipette the hemocytometer pipette is charged with fluid.
- The chamber is then allowed to rest undisturbed for 15-20 min. to allow cells to settle down in moist atmosphere.
- The chamber is then focussed under high power objective of the microscope. The platelets are counted in the central big square (RBC square of area 1 sq mm).
- Platelets appear as bluish bodies, singly or in-groups not > 5 or =5 and are oval, spherical or rod shaped. The platelets can be identified by their highly refractile, silvery appearance which can be revealed by the fine focussing adjustment.

Calculations

Total area counted	:	$1\ mm^2$
Depth of the chamber	:	0.1 mm
Total volume counted	:	area × depth = $0.1\ mm^3$
Let the umber of platelets counted in this area be	:	n
No. of platelets in $1\ mm^3$ of diluted blood	:	n / 0.1
Since dilution is 200 times the number of platelets in $1\ mm^3$ of undiluted blood will be	:	10 n × 200 = 2000 n

Questions:

1. What are the functions of platelets?
2. Enumerate the variations in platelet count.
3. What are the other methods available for platelet count?

13 RETICULOCYTE COUNT

AIM

To count the reticulocytes in a blood smear and to express the relative proportion of these cells to the total number of red cells counted as a percentage.

Theory

Reticulocytes are juvenile RBCs. They are larger then the RBCs (8 μ diameter). They contain remnants of the cytoplasm of the precursor cells like ribosomes and RNA, which have the property of reacting with certain basophilic dyes like brilliant cresyl blue or new methylene blue to form blue precipitates in the form of granules or filaments (reticulum) in unfixed preparations at 37° C.

Materials

- Clean dry glass slides.
- Material for capillary puncture.
- Cedar wood oil.
- Microscope.
- Petridish.
- Filter paper.

Staining of Reticulocytes

- Supra vital stains are used.
- Vital staining is the staining of the cells under natural **living** conditions at 37°C.
- Supravital staining is vital staining of the cells when removed outside the body as in the case of staining of reticulocytes in a blood sample.

Stain consists of:

- *Brilliant cresyl blue / New methylene blue:* 1 gm (stains the basophilic reticulum in cytoplasm).
- *Sodium chloride:* 1 gm (for isotonicity).
- *Sodium citrate:* 3.8 gm (anticoagulant).
- Distilled water to make 100 ml.

Procedure

- Under aseptic precautions a puncture is made on the fingertip with a lancet. First drop of blood is discarded.
- A drop of blood is now placed on a clean glass slide.
- About twice as much of the stain is added and mixed with the blood drop. A coverslip is paced on this mixture. Gentle pressure is exerted to produce a thin film of blood.
- Any excess stain and blood is removed with a filter paper.
- The slide is then kept under a petridish covered with a moist filter paper for about 10-15 minutes, preferably at a temperature of 37° C in a water bath or an incubator. This is to simulate the living conditions, allowing the stain to act on the living cells.
- If incubator is not available then the mixture of blood and twice as much stain is prepared in a test tube and kept in the palm of the hand for 10-15 minutes.
- After gentle shaking of the tube to allow a thorough admixture of the contents a drop of the mixture is placed on a glass slide and a wet film is made as above.
- Alternately, moderately thick smears of this mixture can also be made on glass slides and allowed to dry before microscopic examination.

Observations

Once the wet / dry films are ready they are examined under oil immersion (100 X) objective using cidar wood oil.

Count 500 or 1000 red cells and record the number of reticulocytes (all red cells containing blue staining threads or granules are counted) seen in this cell population as given below. The percentage of reticulocytes is determined.

Field No.	*Number of reticulocytes*	*Number of RBCs*	*Total number of cells*
	(1)	(2)	(1) + (2)
A			
B			
C			
D			

Express the reticulocyte percentage as:

$$\text{Percentage of reticulocytes} = \frac{\text{No. of reticulocytes}}{\text{Total No. of cells counted}} \times 100$$

Questions:

1. What are the normal values of reticulocyte?
2. Name the conditions in which reticulocyte count is high?
3. How do you distinguish a reticulocyte from an RBC and a reticulocyte from a WBC in this experiment?
4. What is the clinical significance of this experiment?
5. Draw a diagram of reticulocyte.
6. Why is the name of the cell as reticulocyte?
7. What is vital, supravital staining how does it differ from Leishman staining?
8. What does the term 'Reticulocytosis' functionally indicate?
9. What stage in erythropoiesis is the reticulocyte?

14 ABSOLUTE EOSINOPHIL COUNT

AIM

To enumerate the number of eosinophils present in 1 cu mm of blood.

Principle

A known amount of capillary blood is diluted with a suitable diluting fluid. The counting chamber is charged with this diluted blood and the eosinophils are counted under the microscope. The absolute count of eosinophils can be calculated from this count and the dilution factor.

Materials

- Haemocytometer.
- WBC pipette.
- Diluting fluid.
- Microscope.
- Petri-dish.
- Materials for capillary puncture.

Diluting Fluid

Pilots Solution: It consists of:

Phloxine	:	1 gm (stains the granules of eosinophils)
Propylene glycol	:	50 ml (vehicle for the stain and lyses RBCs)
Sodium carbonate10%	:	1 ml (accelerates staining)
Distilled water to 100 ml		

Dunger Solution: It consists of:

Aq. Eosin 1%	:	5 ml (stains the granules of eosinophils)
Acetone	:	5 ml (lysis RBCs)
Sodium carbonate 10%	:	1 ml (accelerates staining)
Distilled water to 100 ml		

Procedure

- After taking the usual aseptic precautions, a capillary puncture is made, the first drop of blood is discarded and blood is then drawn upto 0.5 mark of the WBC pipette.
- The diluting fluid is drawn upto the 11 mark and the contents are mixed well for about 2-3 minutes. After discarding 1-2 drops from the pipette, the counting chamber is charged with this fluid mixture.
- The charged chamber is then allowed to stand for 15 minutes under a petri-dish containing moist filter paper. This allows the staining to take place without the evaporation of fluid.
- The eosinophils, which are stained pink to brick red, are counted under the low power of the microscope in the four WBC squares, taking the same precautions as in TLC.
- Morphology of the eosinophils is confirmed under high power.

Calculation: (Similar to TLC)

Let the number of cells in 4 WBCs squares be	:	n
Area of 4 WBCs squares	:	4 sq.mm.
Depth of the chamber	:	0.1 mm
Volume of 4 squares	:	$4 \times 0.1 = 0.4$ cu.mm.
Dilution employed	:	20 times
Number of cells in 0.4 cu.mm. of diluted blood	:	n
Number of cells in 1 cu.mm. of diluted blood	:	n/0.4
Number of cells in 1 cu.mm. of undiluted blood	:	$\frac{n \times 20}{0.4}$

Precautions

1. Eosinophils are confirmed by changing the objective to high power.
2. Other precautions as in TLC.

Questions:

1. What is the normal value of absolute eosinophil count?
2. What are the main functions of eosinophils?
3. Name some conditions where eosinophilia and eosinopenia occurs.
4. Explain the clinical significance of absolute eosinphil count.
5. What happens to eosinophil count in allergic conditions?
6. Name common allergy states where eosinophil count is high?

PART - II

HUMAN EXPERIMENTS

15

RECORDING OF BP AND EFFECT OF POSTURE ON BP

RECORDING OF SYSTEMIC ARTERIAL BLOOD PRESSURE

AIM

To record and interpret blood pressure of the given subject.

Apparatus

An examination couch, sphygmomanometer, stethoscope.

Procedure

Systemic arterial blood pressure can be measured by two methods: Direct and Indirect method.

A. Direct Method

A cannula is introduced into an artery and secured in position with help of ligature, the other end of the cannula is connected to a mercury manometer. This measures the lateral pressure plus the kinetic energy of blood flow at the point of entry cannula (END PRESSURE).

Disadvantage:

This is an invasive procedure and carries the risk of infection.

B. Indirect Method

Principle:

It involves balancing of pressure in a bag i.e. Air pressure against pressure exerted by blood in the artery.

Apparatus:

Sphygmomanometer consists of inflatable flat rubber bag called Riva-Rocci Cuff. The arm bag should be 20% wider than the arm diameter and the length should cover 2/3rd of the arm circumference. The bag is connected by a long rubber tubing to a mercury reservoir on one side and to rubber pump on the other. A small valve regulates the air volume in the bag. The manometer is connected to the mercury reservoir and is U shaped. The graduation is from 0 to 300 mm Hg, with the smallest division corresponding to a reading of 2 mm of Hg.

Procedure

Two methods are commonly in use:

1. Palpatory

i. Ask the subject to sit comfortably on a chair for 5 minutes.
ii. Tie the cuff on the arm about 2.5-3 cm above elbow joint at the heart level.
iii. Feel for the radial pulse and inflate the rubber bag to a pressure to occlude the radial pulse.
iv. Deflate the cuff slowly, releasing the pressure by 2-3 mm Hg/sec; while lowering the pressure, keep palpating the radial artery. Take the reading when the pulse is just felt. This gives the systolic pressure.

Disadvantages

a. Diastolic B.P. cannot be estimated.
b. The systolic pressure is 6-10 mm Hg lower than the pressure measured at the brachial artery by auscultatory method.

2. Auscultatory

i. Ask the subject to sit comfortably on a chair for 5 minutes.
ii. Tie the cuff on the arm about 2.5-3 cm above elbow joint at the heart level.
iii. Place the chest piece of stethoscope over the arm medial to the tendon of biceps where pulsations of brachial artery are felt.
iv. Inflate the cuff rapidly until the pressure in it is well above the systolic blood pressure measured by the palpatory blood pressure.
v. Deflate the cuff slowly, releasing the pressure @ 2-3 mm Hg/sec; while lowering the pressure keep auscultating the brachial artery. Take the reading when a clear tapping sound is heard. This gives the systolic pressure.
vi. The pressure is lowered slowly while listening for the sound of Korotkoff's. The sound becomes dull and muffled. Take the reading when muffling sound is heard. This gives the diastolic pressure.
vii. Take three readings.

Precautions

1. Cuff should be tied over the brachial artery.

2. The cuff should not be either too loosely or too tightly tied.
3. The pressure should fall @ 2-3 mm/Hg/sec. The cuff should not be tied for long periods with raised pressure.

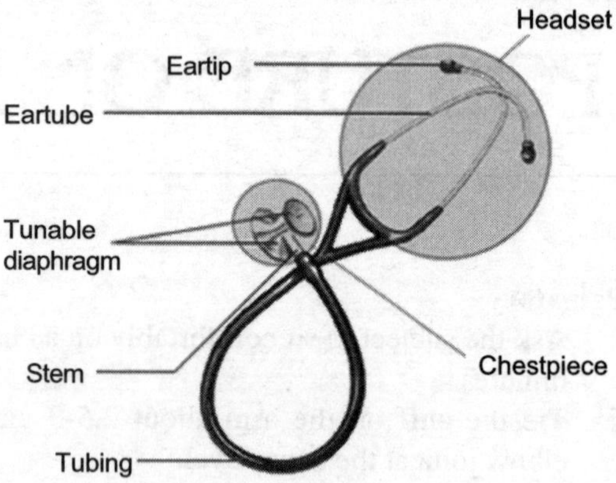

Fig. 15.1

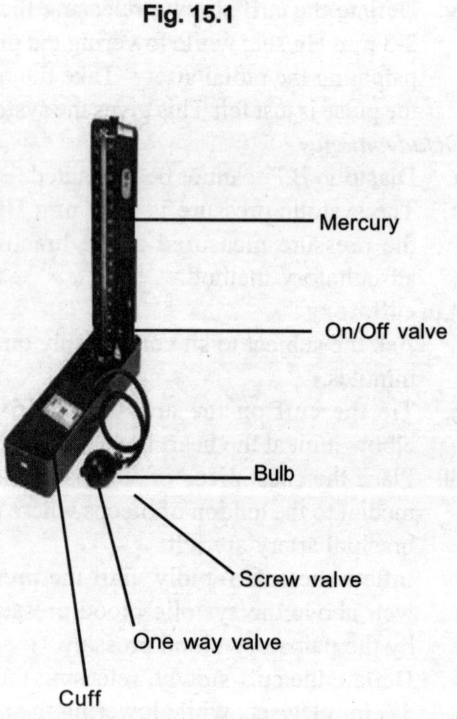

Fig. 15.2

Results and Observations

	Systolic B.P.	*Diastolic B.P.*	*Pulse pressure*	*Mean B.P.*
1st Reading				
2nd Reading				
3rd Reading				

Viva-Voce Questions:

1. Define B.P. What do the diastolic and systolic blood pressure depend upon?
2. What are Korotkoff's sounds? How do they differ from heart sounds?
3. What is auscultatory gap?
4. What are the physiological factors that effect blood pressure?
5. Give the sequence of change in character of Korotkoff's sound when deflating the cuff.

EFFECT OF POSTURE AND EXERCISE ON BLOOD PRESSURE

AIM

To record the effect of posture and exercise on blood pressure.

Apparatus

An examination couch, sphygmomanometer, stethoscope.

A. EFFECT OF POSTURE ON BLOOD PRESSURE

Procedure

1. Ask the subject to lie supine quietly on a couch for 5-10 minutes, record the pulse rate and blood pressure. Do not untie the cuff.
2. Ask the subject to sit up and immediately note the pulse rate and B.P. (by auscultatory method only) every minute for 3-4 minutes.
3. Similarly, make the subject stand from lying position and repeat the whole procedure.
4. Compare the B.P. recorded during the two positions with lying position.

Precautions

1. B.P. should be recorded by keeping brachial artery at heart level in all positions.
2. Since changes in B.P. are sudden, therefore B.P. should be recorded within 30-60 seconds of change of posture.
3. To avoid loss of time, do not untie the cuff.

Observations

Tabulate your result as follows:

Posture	Pulse rate	Systolic/ Diastolic B.P. (mm Hg)	Pulse pressure (mm Hg)
Lying (after 5-10 minutes of rest)			
On sitting			
i. Immediate			
ii. After 2 minutes			
On standing			
i. Immediate			
ii. After 2 minutes			

B. EFFECT OF EXERCISE ON BLOOD PRESSURE

Procedure

1. Allow the subject to sit quietly for 5-10 minutes, take the heart rate (radial pulse) and blood pressure (auscultatory method) and make a note of them.
2. *The exercise:* Various forms of physical activities can be performed as a mode of exercise like climbing upstairs, jumping, hopping, bending etc. The common ones which are used in the laboratory are hop twenty times on each foot, raising the body for 15-20 cm for 3-5 minutes or run up the stairs and back.
3. Immediately after the stoppage of exercise record the heart rate and B.P.
(**Note:** To avoid loss of time, have the sphygmomanometer prepared before exercise with the disconnected cuff in position).
4. The heart rate and B.P. recording should be continued every minute till the resting values are obtained. Note the time of recovery.

Observations

	Heart rate	Systolic/ Diastolic B.P. (mm Hg)	Mean B.P. (mm Hg)	Pulse pressure
1. Resting (after 5-10 minutes of rest)				
2. Immediately after 3 minutes of exercise				
3. Recovery				
2 minutes after exercise				
5 minutes after exercise				

Important Note: In case, the subject feels intolerably breathless, fatigues in legs, giddy or pain, constriction or suffocation in chest during the exercise ask him to discontinue the exercise immediately.

WHO Classification of Grading of Exercise

Grade	*Level*	*Relative load index % of VO_2 max*	*Metabolic (energy) expenditure test (METS)*	*Heart rate*
I	Light	< 25%	<3	<100
II	Moderate	< 50%	<4.5	101-125
III	Heavy	< 75%	<7	125-150
IV	Severe	> 75%	>7	>150

Relative load index is the oxygen consumption as a percentage of VO_2 max. VO_2 max is the maximum oxygen consumption. Metabolic Expenditure Test (METs) is the oxygen consumption in multiples of the basal oxygen consumption.

Viva-Voce Questions:

1. How does the systolic and diastolic blood pressure change with posture? How would you explain these changes in time?
2. How does the heart rate and blood pressure vary with exercise and rest? What may be reason for this variation?
3. What is postural hypotension?

16 MOSSO'S ERGOGRAPHY

AIM

To study the effect of varying load on genesis of fatigue in flexors of middle finger of the given subject by using Mosso's ergograph.

MATERIALS

1. Mosso's ergograph with complete set of weights.
2. Metronome.
3. Paper.
4. Pen marker.
5. Kymograph.

PRINCIPLE

1. *Concept of human fatigue:* Fatigue may be subjective i.e. feeling for a sensation of tiredness or objective i.e. a measurable decrease in performance. These two phenomenons of fatigue are dependent on each other.
2. The development of fatigue in voluntary contracting muscle can be shown by the use of an ergograph in lifting a weight in Mosso's ergograph.

Mosso's Ergograph: Ergograph for isotonic exercise.

It consists of:

1. A *wooden board* fitted with two pairs of *clamps* (curved plates) for fixing the forearm of the subject and a pair of *finger holders* (metal tubes) for fixing the index and ring fingers in position.
2. A *hook* (for suspending weights) attached to a cord, is made to hang over the pulley. The other end of the cord is attached to a *sliding plate*, which moves to and fro.
3. The sliding plate carries a *lever system* to record the movements on a kymograph. The other end of the plate of the plate is connected through a sling to the middle finger of the hand.
4. Alternately, the sliding plate is fitted with a *chart holder*. A pen marker can be fitted vertically over the chart paper so as to record the movements of the chart holder when it moves (Fig. 16.1).

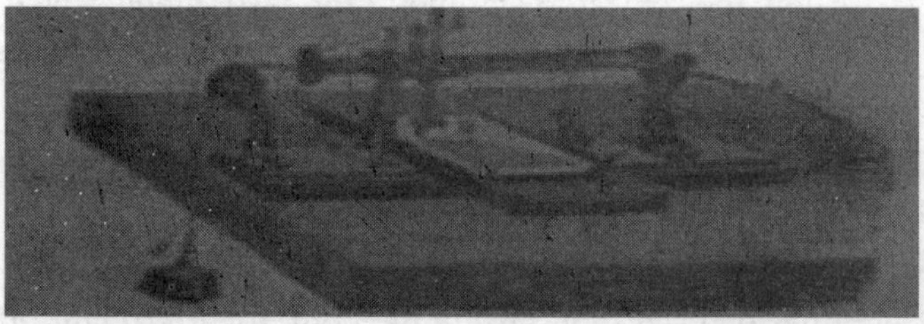

Fig. 16.1

Metronome

It is a timing device, which can be made to beat at definite known intervals.

Procedure

1. The Mosso's ergograph is set on a table of suitable height.
2. Ask the subject to sit comfortably on a stool and clasp the vertical rod with fingers.
3. Fix the arm by tightening the cuffs so as to hold the wrist firmly and ensure movement only of the middle finger.
4. Put a suitable weight usually of 2 kg on the weight stand and adjust the strip of paper and pen marker properly.
5. Set the metronome at 60 per minute. Start the stop watch.
6. Put the middle finger in the sling or hook attached to the string and ask the subject to pull the weight at the rate of 30 per minute till the middle finger is fatigued.
7. Note the duration in seconds of time of onset of fatigue.
8. Ask the subject to take 10 minutes rest.
9. Label the name of the subject, weight used and time of onset of fatigue.
10. Repeat the procedure with 2.5 and 3 kg on the weight stand following the above same steps.

Calculations

Measure the total length of each excursion (D) by adding the peak to peak distance revealed by the lines on the paper. Calculate the work done by the equation.

Work done (W)	=	Force (F) ×	Distance (D)
(kg meters)		(kg)	(meters)

Results

Tabulate your results as follows:

S.No.	*Weight in kg*	*Metronome frequency*	*Fatigue time in min.*	*Work done in kg m.*
1.	2	30/min		
2.	2.5	30/min		
3.	3	30/min		

Obtain the three records and paste them in the file.

Questions:

1. What is fatigue?
2. What is the site of fatigue?
3. What will be the effect of the following factors on the human fatigue during Mosso's ergography?
   (i) Varying the weights to be lifted.
   (ii) Changing the frequency of contractions.
4. How does motivation improve physical performance?

EFFECT OF ARTERIAL AND VENOUS OCCLUSION ON FATIGUE

AIM

To study the effect of arterial and venous occlusion on the onset of fatigue by using Mosso's ergograph.

MATERIALS

1. Mosso's ergograph with weights.
2. Metronome.
3. Paper.
4. Pen marker.
5. Kymograph.
6. Sphygmomanometer.

PRINCIPLE

Blood flow to exercising muscles not only supplies nutrients and oxygen but also removes waste metabolites and heat. Therefore, restricting blood flow to exercising muscles accelerates the onset of fatigue.

a. Venous occlusion by blocking the drainage causes accumulation of waste metabolites in the exercising muscles.
b. Arterial occlusion affects both supply of oxygen and nutrients, and removal of waste metabolites. Therefore, it causes the onset of fatigue early and more effectively.

Procedure

1. The Mosso's ergograph is set on a table of suitable height.
2. Fix the arm by tightening the cuffs so as to hold the wrist firmly and ensure movement only of the middle finger.
3. Suspend a suitable weight usually of 2 or 2.5 kg on the weight stand. Weight should be such that the subject must exert a real effort to lift it up.
4. Set the metronome to 60 per minute and adjust the strip of paper and pen marker properly.
5. Ask the subject to make a series of maximal contractions following the beat of metronome till the middle finger is fatigued.
6. Note the duration in seconds of time of onset of fatigue.
7. Ask the subject to take 10 minutes rest.
8. Wrap the sphygmomanometer cuff round the upper arm of the subject and inflate the cuff to 40 mmHg to occlude venous flow only.
9. Repeat the whole procedure and note the effect of venous occlusion on the time of onset of fatigue
10. Deflate the cuff and ask the subject to rest for 10 minutes.
11. Now raise the pressure of the cuff till the disappearance of the radial pulse (130-140 mmHg) to produce arterial as well as venous occlusion.
12. Repeat the whole procedure and note its effect on the time of onset of fatigue.

Calculations

Measure the total horizontal distance moved till the onset of fatigue labelled as X in each case. As the speed of the drum is 2.5 mm per second so:

2.5 mm distance is covered in................1 sec.
1 mm distance is covered in..................1/2.5 sec.
X mm distance is covered in.................1/2.5x X sec.

Results

Tabulate your results as follows:

S.No.	*Circulation*	*Metronome frequency*	*Weight (kg) constant*	*Onset of fatigue in min*
1.	Intact	30/min		
2.	Venous occlusion	30/min		
3.	Arterial occlusion	30/min		

Obtain the three records and paste them in the file.

Questions:

1. Compare the results of venous occlusion and arterial occlusion on the onset of fatigue.
2. Why fatigue occurs early in arterial occlusion?
3. Name one condition each in which muscle performance gets impaired due to venous occlusion and arterial occlusion.

17 EXAMINATION OF THE RADIAL PULSE

It is always better to feel all the peripheral pulses, but usually radial pulse is the one, which is always felt. It is best felt with the tips of the fingers, the subject's forearm being pronated and slightly flexed. Patient must be fully relaxed before the examination. The following observations should be made.

i. *Rate of Pulse:* Pulse is counted for 1-min. Pulse rate (PR) varies with age: PR=60-100/min in adults and 130-140/min in newborn. Slow pulse < 60/min is called bradycardia and fast pulse > 90/min tachycardia. Pulse rate is increased during exercise, anxiety, fever, and thyrotoxicosis and decreased in myxoedema and incomplete heart blocks.
ii. *Rhythm of Pulse:* Normally the pulse is regular i.e. it beats at a regular interval. Irregular pulse is called arrhythmia. Sinus arrhythmia is increased rate of pulse during inspiration and decreased rate of pulse during expiration. It is a physiological phenomenon caused by change in vagal tone. Irregular rhythm is seen in atrial fibrillation and due to extra-systoles.
iii. *Character of Pulse:* This is most satisfactorily done by palpating a large vessel. Character of pulse takes into account the volume of pulse, its force and tension.
iv. *Volume of Pulse:* By this is meant the amplitude of movement of vessel wall during the passage of the pulse wave. The volume of equivalent pulses on two sides should be compared.
v. *Condition of Vessel Wall:* Sufficient pressure should be exerted on the brachial artery to abolish pulsation in the radial artery, which should be then rolled beneath the fingers against the underlying bones. In young persons, arteries cannot be felt. But in old people they are easily palpable.
vi. *Radio-femoral Delay:* This is examined in the femoral pulses in comparison with the radial by simultaneous examination of the two pulses. The presence or absence, or delay in the femoral pulses in comparison with the radial is noted.

PROFORMA (PULSE EXAMINATION)

Palpable pulsations of carotid in neck:

Radial pulse:

Rate:

Rhythm:

Character:

Volume:

Condition of vessel wall:

Radial-femoral delay:

18 ELECTROCARDIOGRAPHY (ECG)

OBJECTIVES

1. Record and interpret electrocardiogram (ECG) of a normal subject.
2. Calculate heart rate and electrical axis of the heart.

Definitions

Electrocardiogram (ECG) is the graphic record of algebraic sum of action potentials developed during a cardiac cycle and recorded from the body surface. Body is a volume conductor because body fluids are good conductors of electricity therefore electrical changes generated inside the heart with each heart beat are conducted all over the body and can be picked up by means of electrodes placed at certain definite points on the body surface known as leads. Record of these electrical changes during the cardiac cycle is termed Electrocardiogram.

Electrocardiograph is the instrument that can pick up, amplify and record from the body surface the electrical potentials generated by the heart. The instrument should be sensitive to the potential changes of the order of microvolts and have frequency response of 50 to 100 cycles per second.

Electrocardiography is the technique of recording and interpretation of ECG.

Requirements: Electrocardiograph or Physiograph with ECG coupler, Electrodes, Electrode jelly, cables and couch etc.

Recording Conventions

- ECG is recorded on a mm square graph paper, moving at a speed of 25 mm/sec, so 1mm = 0.04 sec (along X axis).
- Amplification settings are selected to get 1mm = 0.1mv on the Y axis. Ideally a potential difference of 1.0 mv should give a deflection of 1.0 cm.
- Any deflection of the record above the base line is regarded as positive deflection and below the base line as negative deflection. No deflection from the base line means isoelectric line or isoelectric segment.
- Spread of excitation towards an electrode gives an upward deflection (positive) and its movement away from it gives a downward (negative) deflection.

Electrocardiograph

The electrocardiograph is an electronic instrument that records and amplifies the difference in electrical potential in any two points on the surface of the body. The earliest type of electronic electrocardiographs used an amplifier driving a cathode ray tube (CRT) the trace being photographed on a moving sensitized paper to provide a permanent record. For direct visual observation Cathode Ray Oscilloscope are used. The time base can be adjusted to one sweep in 5 seconds and a train of several heartbeats can be thus visualized. This form of electrocardiographs is the best option for displaying the ECG to a large group simultaneously. Furthermore, with a double beam CRT heart sound waves can also be displayed at the same time. Since for ECG only 100c/s are required CRT are not used for routine ECG recording, instead a system consisting of an amplifier driving a pen on a moving paper is used.

Information that can be obtained by analyzing ECG:

- The anatomical orientation of the heart.
- The relative size of the chambers.
- Information on heart rate, rhythm and conduction of impulse.
- Types of conduction blocks types and origion of new rhythms (Arrhythmias and extrasystoles).
- Site, duration and extent of ischaemic damage to the myocardium.
- Effects of electrolyte disturbances.
- Influence of certain drugs e.g. digitalis.

Permanent record is available immediately and if desired two or three leads may be recorded simultaneously.

THE LEAD SYSTEMS

Various standard lead systems are used for recording ECG. Each lead is essentially a set of two electrodes, which may be unipolar or a bipolar arrangement of electrode placement. In unipolar recording one electrode is an active or exploring electrode and the other is an indifferent electrode which is kept at zero potential. In bipolar recording both the electrodes are active. Please note that a lead is a combination of two wires and their electrodes to make a complete circuit with the electrocardiograph and not a single wire/electrodes.

Standard Bipolar Limb Leads

These are designated as:

I: Between right arm and left arm.
II : Between right arm and left leg.
III : Between left arm and left leg.

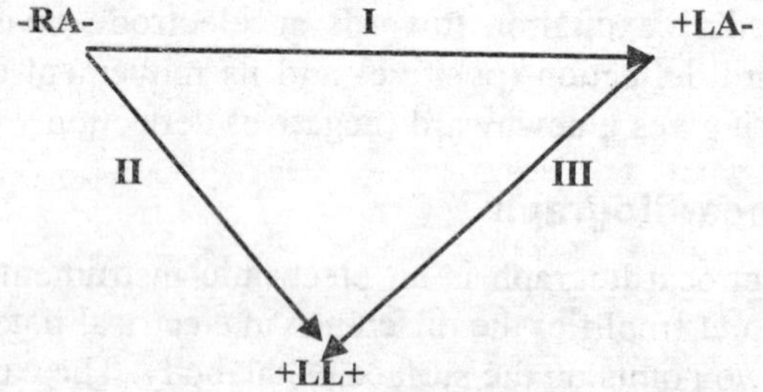

Fig. 18.1

In a volume conductor, the sum of potentials at the points of an equilateral triangle with a current source diapole in the centre is zero at all times. A similar triangle can be approximated in our body by placing electrodes on RA (right arm), LA (left arm) and LL (left leg) with current source as heart in the centre. This is called Einthoven's triangle after the name of the physiologist, Wilhelm Einthoven.

Unipolar Leads

These nine standard locations for placement of unipolar leads are six chest or the pericardial leads are:

V_1 : 4th intercostal space, at the right border of sternum.
V_2 : 4th intercostal space at the left border of sternum
V_3 : midway between V_2 and V_4.
V_4 : 5th intercostal space, mid clavicular line on the left side.
V_5 : 5th intercostal space, anterior axillary line on the left side.
V_6 : 5th intercostal space, mid axillary line on the left side.

The indifferent electrode or zero potential is created by connecting the limb electrode to a common terminal.

The three unipolar limb leads are VR (right arm), VL (left arm) and VF (left foot). The augmented leads designated by the letter 'a' and written as aVR, aVL and aVF are also used when recording is done between one limb and the other two limbs. This arrangement increases the size of the potentials by 50% without any change in the configuration.

PROCEDURE

Using Electrocardiograph

1. Ask the subject to lay supine on the bed comfortably. Make sure he/she has nothing metallic on the body.
2. Check that the instrument is satisfactorily earthed.
3. Apply electrode jelly at the sites if electrode placement. Fix firmly the limb leads marked RA. LA, RL and LL to the respective limbs with the help of rubber straps.
4. Adjust the speed of the chart paper at 25 mm/sec, and obtain a record of caliberation such that 1 mv input gives a 10 mm vertical deflection of the stylus on the chart paper.
5. Adjust the lead selector knob so as to record the activity in lead I,II,III, aVR, aVL and aVF in that order.
6. Apply chest electrodes at the appropriate position on the chest (Fig. 18.2) after applying cardiac jelly; adjust the lead selector knob to chest position and record the activity in chest leads V_1 to V_6 in that order.
7. Label the appropriate strip of the chart paper according to the leads selected.

Alternatively in ECG machine with the provision of automatic recording of all 12 leads, adjust the lead selector to 'auto' position after placing the electrode at appropriate places on the body and take the recording.

Student Physiograph and ECG Coupler

1. Plug in ECG coupler in the consol with consol mains off.
2. Caliberate by taking following steps:
   i. Consol ON, Coupler ON.
   ii. Mode at CAL.
   iii. Select sensitivity of 1 mv on the main amplifier.
   iv. Adjust pen to centre, run paper.
   v. Press cal knob on the coupler slowly (5 sec press release) 3 or 4 times. If amplitude of the cal signal is less or more than 1 cm adjust "GAIN".
3. Connect the Subject through electrode wires to the junction box and connect the junction box to the coupler.
4. Run the paper and take the record at different positions of the lead selector.

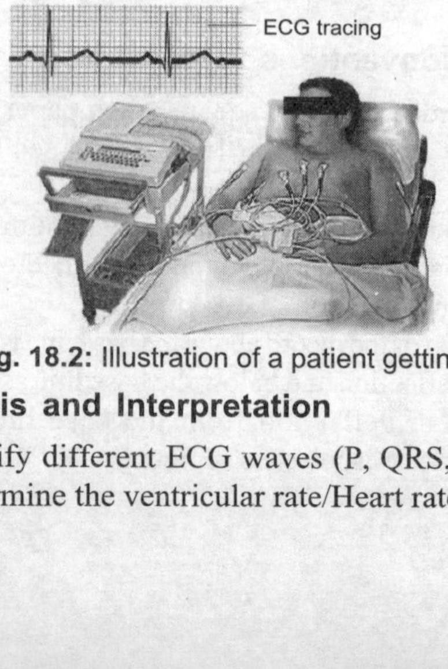

Fig. 18.2: Illustration of a patient getting an ECG

Analysis and Interpretation

1. Identify different ECG waves (P, QRS, T).
2. Determine the ventricular rate/Heart rate and rhythm:

i. May use the formula 1500/RR interval in mm (analyse how?)

ii. For ventricular rhythm measure RR interval in different leads?

3. Similarly, determine atrial rate and rhythm by concentrating on P waves.
4. Tabulate the following:

Form	*Duration*	*Amplitude*	*Remarks*
i. P wave			
ii. QRS complex			
iii. T- wave			
iv. PR interval			
v. OT interval			
vi. ST interval			
vii. ST segment			
viii. T P			

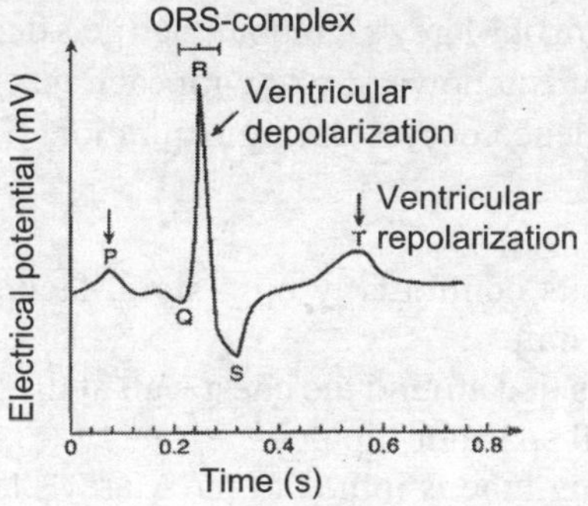

Fig. 18.3

PRECAUTIONS

1. Ensure that the required voltage is available at the mains and the instrument is properly earthed.
2. Subject should be comfortable and should not wear any magnetic/metallic articles, which might interfere with the electric signals of low voltages.
3. Ensure that all leads are in good contact with the body surface.
4. Must check the calibration before taking the record.
5. Use right leg of the subject for grounding the subject for eliminating 50 Hz interference.

Questions:

1. Define Electrocardiogram, Electrocardiography and Electrocardiograph?
2. Why is it necessary to have a recording of 12 leads in electrocardiography? State placement of electrodes in different lead systems.
3. State the purpose of grounding in electrocardiography.
4. State Einthoven's law.
5. State the information you can get from the ECG.
6. Classify main abnormalities of heart action, and how these are reflected in ECG?
7. Which are positive and negative waves of ECG?
8. When will you record a positive or a negative wave or what do you understand by positive or negative wave?
9. What is the pacemaker of the heart?

19 STETHOGRAPHY

AIM

To record movements of chest wall during respiration using stethograph and to record effect of swallowing, sneezing, coughing, speech, hyperventilation and breath holding.

Apparatus

Stethograph, Marey's tambour, Kymograph.

Theory

Stethograph is an instrument for recording the chest wall movements during respiration. The process of recording the respiratory movements is known as stethography. It consists of:

1. *Stethograph:* A corrugated rubber tube 60 cm long and 2 cm in diameter, one and of which is blind and other end is connected through a (pressure) rubber tube to Marey's tambour. A hook and a metallic chain is provided which enables the stethograph to be tied around the chest.
2. *Marey's Tambour:* It is provided with a metallic saucer or cup with its top covered with a latex or rubber diaphragm. To the bottom is a metallic tube, which is connected with stethograph. Thus the pressure variations occurring within the corrugated rubber tube are transmitted to the diaphragm. A marker is placed on the diaphragm to record its movement on kymograph.

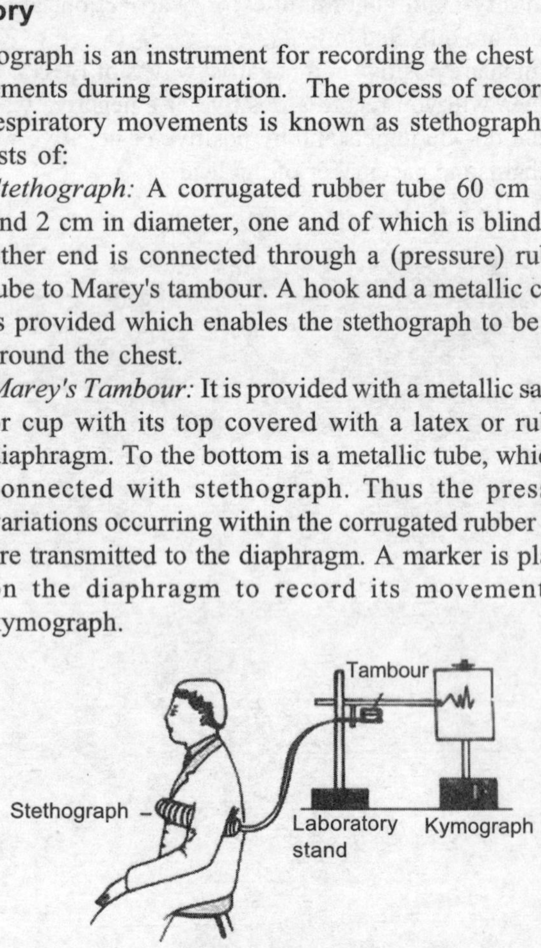

Fig. 19.1

Working

With expansion of chest wall during inspiration, the tube stretches and its volume increases and so the pressure falls.The diaphragm of Marey's tambour then gets depressed and the lever records a down stroke with each inspiration. The opposite sequence occurs during expiration.

Procedure

1. The subject sits comfortably on a stool, facing away from the apparatus.
2. Stethograph is tied around the chest wall at the level of 4th intercostal space or nipples.
3. The connecting tube is joined to the Marey's tambour mounted with a marker on a stand.
4. Marker is made to touch the kymograph, the drum is set to move at a speed of 2.5 mm/sec.
5. Record normal respiratory movements. Note the direction of inspiration and expiration.
6. Note rate of respiration.
7. *Swallowing:* Ask the subject to swallow saliva or a mouthful of water and observe its effect.
8. *Cough:* Ask the subject to cough and observe its effect.
9. *Sneeze:* Ask the subject to sneeze and observe its effect.
10. *Speech:* Ask the student to read aloud from any book or say few words. The voice may be altered in loudness and pitch during the speech. Observe the record any difference.
11. *Voluntary hyperventilation:* Instruct the patient to breathe rapidly and deeply for 15 seconds and then breathe normally. Record the respiration till the normal record is obtained. Ask the subject to take rest for a few minutes before carrying out the next maneuver.
12. *Breath holding:* Ask the patient to hold breath as long as he can after normal inspiration. Record the graph and the duration of breath holding. Ask the patient to hold breath after normal expiration, after deep inspiration and deep expiration. During these maneuvers label the graph for the time and phase of breath in which the respiration was held.

13. *Exercise:* Record normal respiratory movements; stop the drum and with stethograph on his chest the subject exercises by jogging on the same spot for 2 minutes or by running. Start the drum and then ask the subject to hold his breath. Note the effect.

Precautions

1. Check the apparatus for any leaks.
2. Check the rubber tubing for distensibility.
3. Subject should not see the recordings while performing the experiment.
4. The stethograph should be tied snuggly and comfortably.
5. The subject **should not** hyperventilate for more than 30 seconds.
6. Before each record a few normal breaths should be recorded. After the maneuver is performed the drum must be switched off only when the respiration comes back to normal.
7. Record your observations and interpret the results.

Questions:

1. Describe the record obtained during coughing, sneezing and speech. What is the mechanism. How these reflexes are helpful for the body?
2. What is deglutition apnoea? What are the neural pathway involved in this mechanism? How may this be useful for the body? What is aspiration pneumonia?
3. How do the duration of breath holding differ when performed at end of inspiration and expiration. Why may this difference arise?
4. What is breaking point? Why is it caused? What are the levels of pCO_2 and pO_2 at which breaking point may occur normally?
5. Why the person may feel dizzy after 15 to 30 seconds of hyperventilation?
6. Enumerate six important differences between exercise and voluntary hyperventilation?
7. Name the muscles of inspiration/expiration.
8. What is normal rate of respiration?
9. What happens to pCO_2 immediately after hyperventilation?

20

SPIROMETRY

AIM

1. To record the lung volumes and capacities; and
2. To record the vital capacity in different posture.

Requirements

Simple, spirometer and mouthpiece, nose clip, kymograph, Dettol solution, beaker, examination table.

Spirometry is a simple method by which most of the pulmonary volumes and capacities can be measured and the instrument by which this can be done is known as spirometer.

Description of Spirometer

This consists of a bell jar inverted over a chamber of water. The bell-jar is counterbalanced by a weight through a pulley system. Usually atmospheric air is filled in, but the chamber can be filled with oxygen instead of the atmospheric air. A corrugated rubber tube along with a mouthpiece is connected to the inlet. A sodalime chamber can be used over the inlet to record for longer time. **The graph can be recorded by attaching a pen marker and calculations done with the aid of the scale attached to the spirometer**.

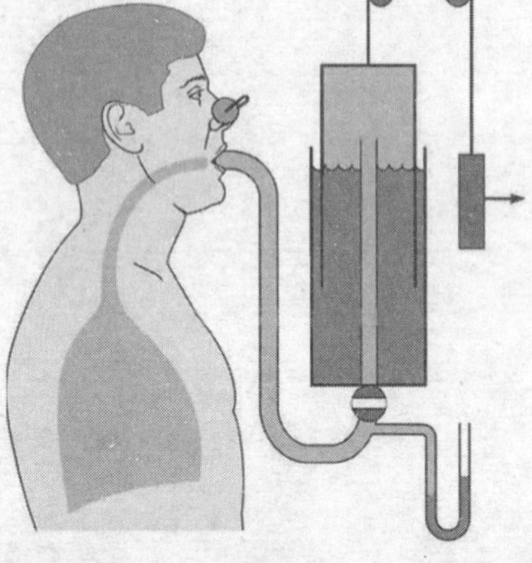

Fig. 20.1

Procedure

The mouth-piece is washed with dettol solution and attached to the rubber tubing. The mouth-piece is taken into the mouth in such a way that two projections should be in between the teeth, the flap should be inside the lips so that there is no leakage from the sides. Nose clip is applied. Drum is rotated at a speed of 2.5 mm/sec. Inspiration is marked upwards and expiration downwards in the recordings. Following volumes and capacities are recorded:

1. **Tidal Volume (TV):** The subject is asked to breathe in and out quietly and the tidal volume is recorded. It is the volume of air inspired or expired with each quiet breath.
2. **Inspiratory Reserve Volume (IRV):** The subject is asked to breathe in maximally following tidal inspiration. The volume of air inspired in excess to tidal inspiration is IRV.
3. **Expiratory Reserve Volume (ERV):** The subject is asked to breathe out maximally following tidal expiration and the volume of air expired in excess to tidal expiration is ERV.
4. **Vital Capacity (VC):** The subject is asked to expire maximally after taking a maximum inspiration. The volume of air expired maximally following a maximal inspiration is **VC=(IRV + TV + ERV)**.
5. **Inspiratory Capacity (IC):** The volume of air that can be inspired maximally at the end of a normal expiration is **IC = (IRV + TV)**.
6. **Maximum Ventilation Volume (MVV):** The subject is asked to breathe in and out as deep and as fast as possible and as long as be can. Routinely the 15 sec duration recording is analyzed and MVV is calculated (1/min).
7. **Respiratory Minute Volume (RMV):** The tidal volume multiplied by respiratory rate gives the RMV (please note that alveolar ventilation is equal to (Tidal Volume – Dead space volume) X Respiratory Rate, and is not synonymous with RMV).

RMV	=	TV × RR (expressed in 1. min)
Breathing Reserve (BR)	=	MVV – RMV
Dyspnoeic Index (DI)	=	$\frac{\text{MVV} - \text{RMV}}{\text{MVV}} \times 100$

The Residual volume (RV), Functional Residual Capacity (FRC) and Total Lung Capacity (TLC) cannot be determined with simple spirometry.

8. **Timed Vital Capacity (TVC) or Forced Expiratory Volume (FEV):** When the expired volume of vital capacity is timed, it is known as timed vital capacity which can be timed for 1st, 2nd and 3rd seconds and represented as FEV_1, FEV_2 and FEV_3 respectively.

To record this, the kymograph is moved at a fast speed of 12.5 mm/sec and the subject is asked to breathe out forcefully and as fast as possible after a maximal inspiration. The volume expired in 1st second is found out and the value expressed as a percentage of vital capacity.

To Record Vital Capacity in Different Postures: The experimental set up is the same as for measuring VC. In addition examination table is required. The subject is asked to breathe out maximally after a maximal inspiration in the following posture (1) Standing; (2) Sitting; and (3) Lying supine.

Questions:

1. Find out the following from your tracings IC, MVV, RMV, BR, DI and FEV_1.
2. What is the difference between static and dynamic lung volumes/capacities?
3. Give the reasons for vital capacity being the lowest in lying position and the highest in standing position.
4. What is the significance of timed vital capacity?
5. What is respiratory dead space?
6. What is dead space hyperventilation?

21 MEASUREMENT OF BASAL METABOLIC RATE (BMR) AND BICYCLE ERGOMETRY

BMR is the energy output of the individual under standardized resting conditions i.e. at complete physical and mental rest 12-18 hours after a meal (post-absorptive period) and in an equable environmental temperature. Clinically the BMR is expressed as a percentage above or below the accepted normal standard taking into account the age, height, body weight etc.

BENEDICT-ROTH METHOD

Requisites

Spirometer with a soda-lime chamber or the Benedict-Roth apparatus for determining oxygen consumption, couch, oxygen cylinder, nose clip, dettol, cotton, barometer, thermometer, height and weight measuring equipment, charts for correction of gas volumes, Mayo's tables and Dubois nomograms for normal BMR values and for finding body surface area.

I. PROCEDURE

Preparation of the Subject:

1. **To Keep the Subject in Post Absorptive State:** Since the investigation is to be carried out in post absorptive state (i.e. 12-18 hours after the last meal), it is customary to give the subject a meal (preferably less in proteins) the previous night and to carry out the estimation in the next morning.
2. **To Ensure Complete Physical and Mental Rest:**
   - i. The subject should have had a restful sleep the previous night.
   - ii. He is not subjected to any physical and mental stress. He is normally transported by a wheel chair or stretcher to the place of investigation.
   - iii. Subject is allowed to rest (preferably in the lying position for a minimum of 30 min prior to the investigation).
   - iv. He is shielded from all environmental stimuli and causes of anxiety. It is sometimes necessary to emphasise the harmless nature of the test itself to the subject. But the subject is not allowed to sleep during the investigation.

Indirect Calorimetry

Principle

All commonly used clinical forms of basal metabolism employ the indirect principle, wherein oxygen consumption is measured and translated into terms of heat production.

Steps

1. Note the temperature and the barometric pressure. Record the height (cm) and weight (kg) and note age and sex of the subject.
2. Fill the bell of the apparatus with 100% O_2.
3. Connect the subject to the apparatus through the mouthpiece and clip the nose. By adjusting the two-way tap, allow the subject to breathe from the atmosphere for a few minutes.
4. Then turn the tap and connect the subject to the spirometer so that he inspires O_2 from the bell and expires air into the spirometer. CO_2 is removed by soda lime contained in the inner part of the spirometer. The kymograph is simultaneously started.
5. As oxygen is consumed the bell is lowered and simultaneously tracing of respiratory movements is recorded on the moving drum.

II. CALCULATIONS

A. Calculations of Oxygen Consumption Per Minute (From Record Obtained)

$$O = \frac{(\text{Initial level of } O_2 - \text{Final level of } O_2) \text{ after 6 minutes}}{6}$$

B. Calculation of BMR

1. Volume of O_2 consumed per minute at BTPS = 'O' liters.

2. O_2 consumed at 1 hour or 60 minutes = 60.0 liters at BTPS.
3. Convert O_2 level at BTPS to STP using correction factor "C" from tables.
4. Corrected volume of O_2 consumed at STP in one hour = 60.O.C liters.
5. Therefore, heat liberation in one hour = 60.O.C × 4.875 liters.
(Where 4.875 kcal is the calorific value of one liter of O_2 consumed per hour at STP).
6. Find out the body surface area (BSA) in sq. meters from the Dubois normogram or by using.

Dubois formula

$$\text{BSA in } m^2 = W^{0.425} \times H^{0.725} \times 71.84$$

Where W is the weight of the subject in kg and H is the height in cm.

7. The BMR of the subject $= \frac{60.\text{O.C.} \times 4.875}{\text{BSA}}$ Kcal/m²/hour
8. Find out the **expected BMR** for the Mayo's table according to the age and sex of the subject.
9. Determine the percentage difference from accepted **Expected** standard

i.e. percentage BMR $= \frac{\text{Calculated BMR-Expected BMR}}{\text{Expected BMR}} \times 100$

Normal Value

The BMR of an adult between the ages 25-50 years is about 40-37 Cals/hr/m². The normal range of percentage change is 15.

Viva-Voce Questions:

1. What are the various factors affecting basal metabolic rate? How do these affect the basal metabolic rate?
2. What is the normal body surface area?
3. What are the precautions to be taken before carrying out the basal metabolic experiment?
4. What is the clinical significance for measuring basal metabolic rate?
5. Name the conditions causing increase or decrease in BMR.

BICYCLE ERGOMETERY

AIM

To find out energy cost of work and determine mechanical efficiency with the help of a bicycle ergometer.

APPARATUS

Spirometer with a soda lime container and a recording kymograph or Benedict Roth apparatus for determining oxygen consumption, oxygen cylinder, nose clips, mouth piece, Dettol, cotton, barometer, height and weight measuring equipment, bicycle ergometer, stethoscope, thermometer, metronome, B.P. apparatus, measuring tape, stop watch.

BICYCLE ERGOMETER

It is in the form of a bicycle with the frame fixed to a board. It has only the rear wheel, the dimensions of which are:

Radius	-	27 cm
Diameter	-	54 cm
Circumference	-	169.7 cm

The rear wheel has a strong tape passed over the rim. At the free ends, the tape is connected to two spring balances (T_1 and T_2) and these can monitor the force against which the subject pedals. The force is kept constant for one set of readings. The difference in the spring balance readings measures the tension in the tape (T_1-T_2). A counting device is connected to the rear wheel so that the number of revolutions can be directly read.

PROCEDURE

1. Note the room temperature and the barometric pressure, age, sex, weight (kg) and height (cm) of the subject.
2. Note the heart rate, blood pressure and the respiration rate of the subject.
3. Allow the subject to rest on a couch for 10-15 minutes before the test.
4. Fill the bell of the apparatus with 100% O_2 and ask the subject to sit on the bicycle ergometer.
5. Connect the subject to the spirometer through the mouthpiece and clip the nose. By adjusting the two-way tap, allow the subject to breath from the atmosphere for a few minutes.
6. Start the drum and turn the tap thereby connecting the subject to the spirometer so that he inspires O_2 from the bell and expires air into the spirometer. CO_2 is removed by the soda lime contained in the inner part of the spirometer.
7. As oxygen is consumed the bell is lowered and the recording keeps going up with simultaneous recording of the respiratory movements on the moving drum. Calculate the resting oxygen consumption (O_R) from the graph obtained just as it is measured in the BMR experiment.
8. Disconnect the subject from the spirometer. Again fill the bell with 100% oxygen.
9. After a short period, adjust the metronome to 50-60 beats per minute and ask the subject to pedal the bicycle at the same rate i.e. his feet push the pedal to each beat of the metronome. The rate can be varied to any that is optimum for the subject being tested and metronome adjusted accordingly.

10. Adjust the **tension load (breaking resistance T_1-T_2 i .e. difference between the spring balances)** at 2 kg; set the counting device at zero reading and ask him to respire from the mouth piece which is connected to the atmosphere. Measure the heart rate, respiratory rate and blood pressure as he pedals for 5-6 minutes.
11. When three readings of heart rate/ respiratory rate/ blood pressure are stabilized or consistent, the subject is said to have reached a steady state and is then connected to the spirometer and he continues to pedal for the next 4-6 minutes with simultaneous recording of respiratory movements.
12. The O_2 consumption during exercise (O_E) is calculated from the graph obtained. The tension is measured by noting the difference in readings of the two spring balances. The distance moved is calculated by noting the circumference of the wheel and the number of revolutions made by him.
13. Allow the subject to recover and note his heart rate, respiratory rate and blood pressure during recovery at 2 minutes and 5 minutes after stoppage of exercise.

CALCULATIONS

Efficiency is expressed by the formula:

$$\text{Efficiency (\%)} = \frac{\text{Work done (W)}}{\text{Energy used }(E_W - E_R)} \times 100 \text{ or } \frac{\text{Output}}{\text{Input}} \times \frac{100}{(O_R - O_E) \times 4.875}$$

E_R: Energy consumed during work O_R= O_2 consumed during rest

E_W: Energy consumed at rest O_E= O_2 consumed during exercise

- **Calculations of Oxygen Consumption Per Minute at BTPS**

  The slope of a line joining the ends of each of the spirometer excursions on the graph obtained is proportionate to the O_2 consumption. Such a line is drawn on the graph obtained.

  The amount of O_2 (in milliliters) consumed per minute can be obtained by dropping 2 perpendiculars from the baseline onto the slope (in the uniform portion of the graph). Note the initial and the final volume of O_2 consumed.

Volume of O_2 consumed per minute at BTPS = 'O' liters.

$$\text{“O”} = \frac{\text{Final level of } O_2 - \text{ Initial level of } O_2}{\text{Time in min}} \text{ liters/min}$$

Both the resting oxygen consumption and the O_2 consumption during exercise are calculated by the above formula.

- **Convert O_2 Level at BTPS to STP Using Correction Factor “C” from Tables**

  O_R = O_2 (liters) consumed/min during resting conditions.

  O_E = O_2 (liters) consumed/min during exercise.

- **Calculation of Work Done (W)**

Work done (W)(kgm) = Distance (m) × Force (kg)

= Distance × breaking resistance ($T_1 - T_2$)

= Wheel circumference × r.p.m.× Tension (kg)

$$= \frac{2\Pi m}{100} \text{ (meters)} \times \text{Tension (kg)}$$

where r is the radius of the wheel of the bicycle in cm and n is the number of revolutions per min (Counter reading Total exercise time in minutes)

= Work done in kgm/min

- **Calculation of Mechanical Efficiency**

$$\text{Mechanical efficiency} = \frac{\text{Output}}{\text{Input}} \times 100$$

The work done (Output) and energy used (Input) must be expressed in the same units.

Following conversions may be applied:

- **For Work Done (Output)**

  1 k cal =426.7 kgm

  Calculate work done in kgm/min

  And convert into k cal/min **(Output)**

- **For Energy Consumed (Input)**

  1 liter of O_2 consumed = 4.875 kcal

  Calculate O_2 consumption per min during resting (basal) conditions O_R

  Calculate O_2 consumption per minute during exercise O_E

  Oxygen consumed for the work or exercise= O_E-O_B

  Convert O_E-O_B into Kcal = (O_E-O_B) × 4.875 **(Input)**

$$\text{Mechanical efficiency} = \frac{\text{Output}}{\text{Input}} \times 100$$

Precautions

- Make sure that there is no leak (of air) from the spirometer and from mouthpiece.
- The subject should not be facing the spirometer while recording the oxygen consumption.
- Soda lime should be fresh and filled to about 2/3rd of the cylinder.
- Ensure the steady state of the subject during exercise before recording oxygen consumption.
- The subject should pedal as close to the frequency of metronome.
- Set the counting device at zero reading before starting exercise.
- For mechanical efficiency the exercise should be of moderate severity (O_2 consumption 1-1.5 lit/min).

Questions:

1. What is steady state exercise?
2. How would you classify exercise?
3. What do you mean by treadmill test?
4. Define O_2 debt and O_2 deficit.

22

CARDIAC EFFICIENCY TEST

These tests are based on the response of CVS to a standardized exercise to which the body is subjected. With an efficient cardiovascular functioning there is prompt response to a sudden stress e.g. exercise but the increase in heart rate and BP is minimal. At the end of this period of stress or exercise the heart rate and BP soon return to the resting level. The response to exercise depends on cardiac reserves, nutrition, skill, muscle power and motivation of the person.

It is one of the tests for physical fitness. In order to establish a clinical standard of cardiac efficiency it is necessary to adopt a definite amount of work as test, to be applied to the heart under examination, and this is best done by formulating a standard exercise performed by a subject. During and after this performance, observations are made which serve as an index to the efficiency of heart.

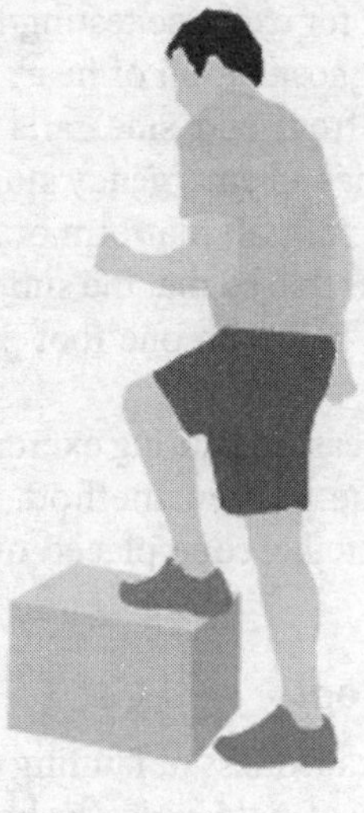

I. Harward's Step Test:

Ht. of Step – 18"

Ask the subject to take vigorous exercise of 20 steps/ min. for a period of 5 minutes so that at the end of it, he feels completely exhausted. In case the subject is unable to continue the test for 5 minutes, he may perform the test for a shorter period of time.

Record the pulse after the exercise at the following intervals.

a. After 1 minute to 1 minute 30 seconds.
b. After 2 minutes to 2 minutes 30 seconds.
c. After 4 minutes to 4 minute 30 seconds

$$\text{Then efficiency index} = \frac{\text{Duration of exercise in sec.}}{2(a+b+c)} \times 100$$

In normal individuals, it is 100% but it is more in athletes.

Interpretation of scores is as follows:

Above 90= Excellent
80-90= Good
55-70= Average
Below 55= Poor physical condition

II. Master's Step Test

Note the basal pulse rate of the person. Ask to step up and down the platform (Ht. 9", depth 10" and width 27") 12 times per minute. Note his pulse rate immediately after the exercise is over. Note the recovery time for pulse rate to come to normal level.

Repeat the experiment by increasing frequency of steps to 18, 24 and 30 per minute. And note the pulse rate after each exercise and recovery time for pulse rate to come to normal. In normal person the pulse rate after exercise should return to initial value in 5 minutes.

Other Tests

- Treadmill test.
- Bicycle ergometry.

Questions:

1. What is the cardiac reserve?
2. What are your observations? Comment on the fitness of your subject.

23 TREADMILL TEST

The major indications for exercise testing by the treadmill are diagnosis and prognostication of heart disease.

The treadmill has front and side rails for subjects to steady themselves. It has an emergency stop button readily available for the staff. A small platform or stepping area at the level of belt is advisable so that the subject can start the test by "pedaling" the belt with one foot prior to stepping on.

Blood pressure is measured during exercise by automatic means or by the time-proven method of holding the subject's arm with a stethoscope placed over the brachial artery.

Pretest Requirements

- History of light-headedness or fainting during exercise, and family history of sudden death should be verified.
- Subject is neither to eat nor smoke at least 2 hours prior to the test.
- Acute MI, arrhythmias, unstable angina need to be ruled out by history and physical examination (especially noting systolic murmurs).
- Take drug history for e.g. β-blockers as they should not be stopped before testing as cardiac abnormalities surface.
- Pretest standard 12-lead ECG in both supine and standing positions is necessary to record the baseline.

During the Test

- Target heart rates under supervision are attained.
- The test is stopped if a drop in systolic BP, anginal chest pain, signs of poor perfusion (pallor, cyanosis) or ECG changes of ST depression or elevation appear.

After Exercise

- The patient walks down slowly to delay the appearance of any ST segment abnormalities during recovery.

Bicycle Ergometry Vs Treadmill

The bicycle ergometry is cheaper, makes less noise and occupies less space. The only disadvantage is that the pedaling speed needs to be maintained essentially the same.

The automated bicycle ergometers that do are very costly. The upper body motion is reduced in the bicycle ergometer.

The treadmill test is purely for the patients who prefer walking to cycling. Upper body motion is also used. The bicycle ergometer may be substituted for the treadmill for measurements of V_{O_2MAX}.

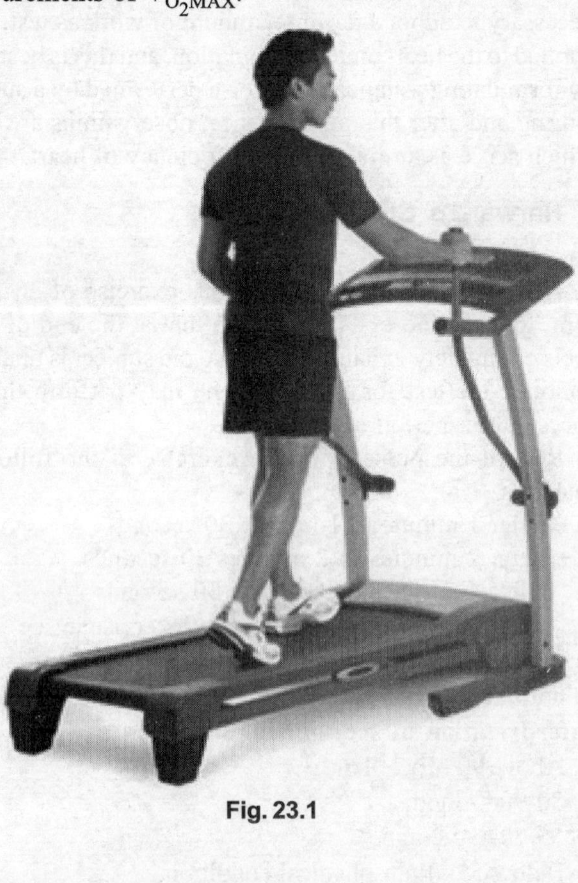

Fig. 23.1

24 PREGNANCY DIAGNOSTIC TEST

AIM

To detect pregnancy in its very early stages.

Principle

The pregnancy diagnostic tests depend on the presence of human chorionic gonadotropin (HCG) in the urine of the pregnant woman.

Tests

Principle: The tests for pregnancy diagnosis are of two types: immunologic and biologic. The biologic ones are more sensitive but no longer done. In this the human pregnant urine is injected in an animal and the effect of HCG on their reproductive organs and ovulation status is observed. Examples are the Aschheim-Zondek test, the Friedman test and the Galli-Mainini test.

The immunologic test, which is mostly used, is the Gravindex Test. The Gravindex kit consists of Gravindex antigen (latex particles coated with HCG), Gravindex antibody (serum containing HCG antibodies), dark slide, sticks and a pipette. In this test, an early morning sample of urine is taken and mixed with Gravindex antigen and Gravindex antibody. If there is agglutination, then pregnancy is generally ruled out. Absence of agglutination suggests pregnancy.

The principle of the above test is as follows: If antibodies to HCG are allowed to react with HCG-coated red cells or latex particles, agglutination of the red cells or latex particles occurs. But if the antibodies are allowed to react with urine containing HCG prior to the reaction with red cells or latex particles, there is no agglutination of red cells or latex particles, since HCG of the urine has consumed the antibodies.

Questions:

1. Describe your observations with the help of a labelled diagram.
2. When can this test be false-positive?
3. What is the other clinical condition in which this test can be useful?

25 PERIMETRY

AIM

To chart the peripheral field of vision and the blind spot.

REQUISITES

Perimeter and its accessories.

Theory

The peripheral field of vision of an eye is the extent of the external world, which is seen by the eye at any given moment. It is the sum of the objects that form images upon the retina when the gaze is fixed at a particular point.

Perimetry is the term applied to the procedure of mapping out the visual fields, using a perimeter.

Peripheral field of vision is the peripheral (outer) limit of the field of vision. The visual field is not circular as its extent is limited by the nose medially, orbit above and cheek below.

Blind spot or physiological scotoma: This is an area located in the temporal quadrant of the visual field in which there is no perception of light. This corresponds to the optic disc i.e. the small area of retina where optic nerve leaves the eye. It contains no light sensitive receptors (rods and cones) and thus vision is not possible over this area. This area is therefore called the blind spot.

Binocular vision: The two visual fields, one for each eye, overlap in the medial part forming the so called area of binocular vision in which can object is seen by both eyes. It plays an important role in appreciation of depth and proportion of objects.

PROCEDURE

Although, precise charting of the field of vision requires a perimeter, a crude idea of the field of vision can be obtained using the Confrontation method in common clinical practice.

Confrontation Method

Seat yourself opposite to the subject at a distance of about ½ metre (arms length) from him. Test both eyes separately. If the right eye is to be tested, ask the subject to close the left eye (by cupping with his hand), and look steadily at your left eye. Look steadily yourself at the subject's right eye, your own right eye being closed. Now hold your left hand far out, midway between the subject and you, and keep moving the index finger. Ask him to say "yes" as soon as he perceives the moving finger. You then compare the position at which you first see your finger with that at which the subject sees it first, assuming that your field of vision is normal. The procedure is repeated in various directions. The left eye of the subject can be tested in the same way using your right hand.

Perimetry

Perimeter:

- The perimeter consists of a **rotating arc** easily revolved around a pivot on a vertical stand.
- The arc can be rotated in any direction and can also be fixed at any position with the help of a tightening screw.
- The arc is **graduated from 0° to 90°,** the "zero" being at the center and the 90° at the periphery.
- The center of the arc i.e. point of pivot, is occupied by a white disc 5 mm in diameter. This is the **fixation point** and the subject is asked to fix the gaze at it while the field of vision is being mapped out.
- The arc bears a moveable **test object.** The colour (white, yellow, blue, red and green), shape (square, circle) and size of the object can be varied. It can be moved along the length of the arc from its periphery to the center.
- An adjustable **chin rest** is fixed in front of the arc. It has two chin cups. The right chin cup is used for mapping the visual field of the left eye and vice versa.
- A **detachable fixation rod** is provided in front of the chin rest.
- Behind the arc, there is a **holder for the perimeter chart.** It has a central pin, which pierces the center of the chart paper when the chart is fixed to this holder.

It also has a **metallic graduated scale** with a moveable **punch marker.** It is used to punch mark degrees on the perimeter chart paper, in accordance with the position of the object on the arc while testing.

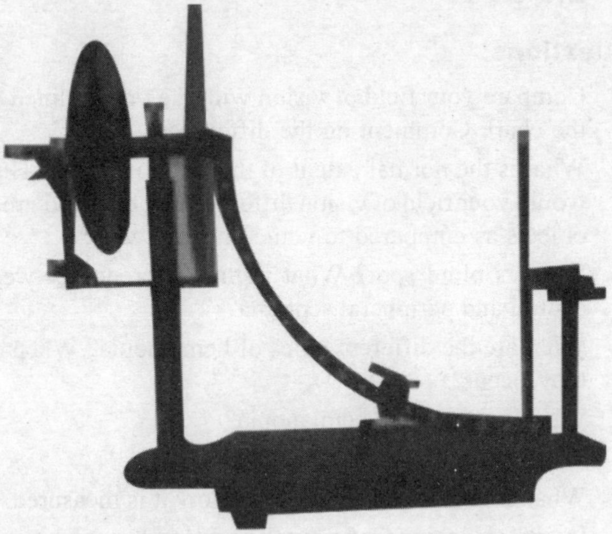

Fig. 25.1: Showing Lister's perimeter

The Perimeter Chart

- Shows concentric circles at intervals of 10° from 10° to 90° called **isopters.**
- The centre point of the chart corresponds with the visual axis and the fixation point. Therefore, all the points on a particular concentric line **(isopter)** subtend the same visual angle with the visual axis at the nodal point of the eye.
- The radii of the circles are marked at 15° intervals, which denote the various **meridians.**
- The two normal visual fields are marked on the chart.
- Two circles one on the right side and one on the left side, marked on the horizontal meridian at 15°, represent the blind spots of each eye as determined by the scotometer and not the perimeter.
- The chart is attached to the back of the perimeter and it rotates with the arc.
- The position of the object is marked in degrees on the chart using the isopters while the meridians are used to move the arc by 15° each time.

Fixing the Perimeter Chart

Fixing the perimeter chart is same for both eyes.

- Place the metallic arc in the horizontal position (90° meridian) on the right side of the subject, i.e. in the right temporal field.
- The chart paper is then fixed upright at the back of the perimeter in the chart holder with the central pin piercing the center point of the innermost circle of the chart paper and the 90° meridan lying horizontal, in line with the scale of the punch marker (i.e. the punch marker should move on this meridian).
- Ensure that the visual field marked on the chart and offered to the punch marker corresponds with the subject's field of vision being tested.

Positioning of Subject

One eye is to be tested at a time.

- Ensure illumination is adequate and if the subject wears spectacles, they should be removed, as the frame will restrict the visual field.
- Seat the subject comfortably in front of the apparatus and ask him to rest chin on the appropriate chin rest (use the right chin rest for testing the left eye and vice versa).
- The fixation rod is used to adjust the level of the chin rest and hence the level of the eye of the subject. The fixation rod is put into its slot in front of the chin rest with the subject resting his chin on it. The height of the chin rest is so adjusted that the pupil of the eye of the subject is in line with the top (white part) of the rod and hence the fixation point of the perimeter. The rod is then removed.
- The subject covers his other eye by cupping his hand over it and fixes his gaze on the central fixation point. **Instruct him not to shift his gaze from the fixation point during testing.**

Object Used

- Normally, charting is done with a white object of standard 7 mm size square. If the subject's vision is poor then a larger 10 mm size square can be used.

Charting the Peripheral Field of Vision

- The observer stands behind the perimeter so that he does not come in the field of vision of the subject during testing.
- The rotating arc is kept in a particular meridian and the object is moved from the end of the arc towards fixation point, till it is just perceived by the eye (as a white blur). The subject says "yes" and that particular point is noted on the chart for that particular meridian.
- Move the target object further throughout the length of the arc upto the fixation point in order to detect any blind spot within the field of vision.
- Repeat the whole procedure at 15° intervals (24 meridans) till the field of vision is marked in the four quadrants.
- The peripheral field of vision is plotted by joining the 24 points altogether.
- Similarly test the other eye.

Mapping of Blind Spot

- Fix the metallic arc in the 90° horizontal meridian in the temporal field of vision of the eye to be tested, as the blind spot is perceived in the respective temporal field.
- In this meridian and in 2 or 3 meridians below it (each less than 5° apart) if the movement of the object is continued after it is perceived, at a particular point it will disappear from the field and on further movement, will reappear in the field. The subject is asked to indicate both disappearance and reappearance of the object and these points are marked on the chart. A circle joining all these points gives the blind spot for that visual field.

Maping the Field of Vision for Coloured Objects

- The test object has other colours like blue, red and green. Using the 7 mm square size these objects can be used to map the field of vision for various colours just the same way as the white object.
- Plot the field of vision using blue, red and green coloured objects and compare with that plotted with the white object.

Labelling the Chart

Indicate on the chart:

- Name, age and sex of the subject.
- Size (in mm), shape and colour of the test object.
- Eye tested.

Questions:

1. Compare your field of vision with the one outlined on the chart. Comment on the differences, if any.
2. What is the normal extent of the field of vision? How would your field of vision differ for red, blue and green objects as compared to white one and why?
3. What is blind spot? What is the difference between central and peripheral scotoma?
4. What are the different types of hemianopia? When do they occur?
5. What is anopia and hemianopia?
6. What are the types of hemianopia?
7. What is central field of vision? How it is measured?
8. In which lesions of visual pathways, perimetry is clinically used?

26 OPHTHALMOSCOPY, AMBLYOSCOPY, TONOMETRY, COLOUR VISION AND RETINOSCOPY

OPHTHALMOSCOPY

Ophthalmoscopy is essential part of complete medical examination.

Give useful information regarding optic nerve head, local ophthalmic conditions.

It is useful as a preliminary examination to diagnose certain diseases, as it gives information regarding hypertensive retinopathy, diabetic retinopathy and other systemic ailments.

Requisites

2% Homatropine (Cycloplegic), Indirect ophthalmoscope, Direct ophthalmoscope.

Apparatus and Instrument

The Ophthalmoscope (invented by Hermann von Helmoltz in 1950)

An ophthalmoscope consists of the following components:

1. **The handle:** It possesses three mirrors and also serves as a case for dry cells.
2. The three mirrors are two concave (one large and one small) and one plane.
   i. The **large concave** mirror is used for indirect ophthalmoscopy and the smaller one for direct ophthalmoscopy.
   ii. The plane mirror is used for retinoscopy.
   iii. Each mirror is having a central aperture, called sight hole or viewing aperture. It is placed just above a system of prisms which reflects parallel beam of light from a low voltage bulb.
   The aperture is divided into two parts:
      a. Lower half for throwing light into the subject's eye; and
      b. Upper half for the examiner's observation.
3. **Serrated (or notched) disc:** It contains series of lenses. The disc can be rotated to move the desired lens against the viewing aperture. The diopteric power of the lens in use is indicated on the back of the instrument.
4. **On/Off switch:** By rotating this ring, the amount of light being directed into the subject's eye can be controlled.

Important Note: If the examiner himself has any refractive error, he should use his glasses while using the ophthalmoscope).

Procedure

To be conducted in three steps:

1. Preliminary examination with plane mirror at 1 meter.
2. Indirect ophthalmoscopy.
3. Direct ophthalmoscopy.

Subject taken to dark room for ophthalmoscopy. Subject should be lying/sitting. Subject and observer relax their accomodation. Subject is asked to gaze at distant object to relax accommodation. Then conduct preliminary/ indirect ophthalmoscopy and direct ophthalmoscopy.

Preliminary Examination: Like retinoscopy and give information about refractory status of the eye, opacities.

Direct Ophthalmoscopy: This makes use of the ophthalmoscope. It is self-illuminated instrument with an aperture for observation. It has a series of lens of various focal lengths, which can be moved into the line of vision while examination is being performed.

Important Viva-Voce Questions:

1. Give the differences between indirect and direct ophthalmoscopy.
2. What information can be obtained by ophthalmoscopy?
3. What is physiological cup?
4. Describe ophthalmoscopic features of the normal retina.

Examination of the fundus of the eye with the help of an ophthalmoscope is an essential part of every complete medical examination. Valuable information may be obtained as to the state of optic nerve head and local ophthalmic conditions.

In routine medical examination it is usually possible with practice to examine the optic disc and surrounding retina without dilating the pupil. For complete examination of the fundus, dilation of the pupil is a must and can be done by adding a few drops of 2% Homatropine into the conjunctival sac. There are two ways by which the ophthalmoscopy can be performed: (1) Indirect Method (2) Direct Method.

For both the methods the examination is done in a dark room with the patient either in the sitting or lying down. Both the subject and the observer should relax their accommodation by looking into the distance in spite of the fact that the object looked at is only a few inches away. Both must remove spectacles if worn. Use the right eye to look at the subject's right eye and the left eye to look at his left eye.

1. **The Indirect Method:** Here, a concave mirror with a central sight hole is used. The observer sits in front of the subject at arms length. The light is focussed to the eye of the subject and a +13 D lens is interposed to make the subject's eye highly myopic. The observer moves forwards or backwards until the fundus is sharply focussed. A real magnified and inverted image of the fundus is formed between the observer and the lens. The image is magnified 5 times.
2. **Direct Method:** This makes use of the ophthalmoscope. It is a self-illuminated instrument with an aperture for observation. It has a series of lens of various focal lengths, which can be moved into the line of vision while the examination is being performed.

   Ask the subject to keep his eye fixed on some suitable object and relax his accommodation. Then begin at arm length from the subject and near his line of sight, look through the aperture of the ophthalmoscope while studying it against the bridge of your nose and shine the beam on to the subject's eye. A glow from the pupil is now seen. It is known as the **red reflex.** Now bring the ophthalmoscope as close as possible to the patient's eye and direct the light slightly nasally. In this way the optic disc can be found and the light will not shine directly on the macula. If the optic disc is not in focus reduce the strength of the lens gradually until the disc becomes sharply focussed. If the observer's eye is emmetropic and his accommodation is relaxed the strength of the lenses necessary to bring the fundus into focus gives an indication of the refractory error of the subject's eye. The magnification by this instrument is 15 times.

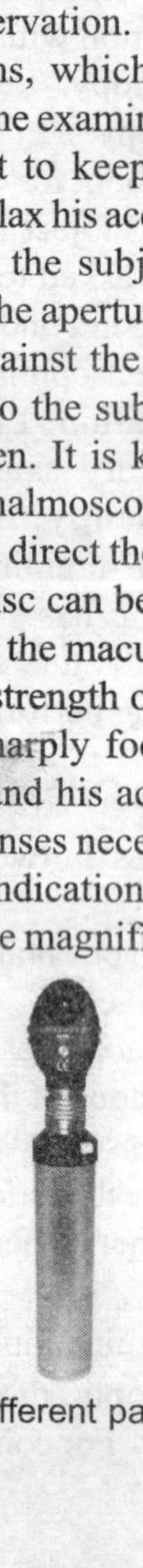

Fig. 26.1: Label the different parts of ophthalmoscope

Questions:

1. Draw the normal fundus.
2. What information may you receive from observing the normal fundus?
3. What are important indications for indirect ophthalmoscopy?

AMBLYOSCOPY

Amblyoscopy is the technique with which the grades of binocular vision can be assessed with the amblyoscope. Amblyoscopy is also employed as one of the orthoptic exercises to improve the stereoscopic vision.

Procedure

The grades of binocular vision may be detected by using a stereoscope or its more adaptable development the amblyoscope. Amblyoscope has two adjustable tubes each of, which carries a picture, which is presented to one eye. The subject then moves the two tubes either towards each other or away from each other until he is able to perceive the two pictures as one. The degree to which the two tubes are separated may be taken as a measurement of the development of the fusion facility (normally occurs between 0-15°). It can also be assessed if the person is able to fuse the images and maintain for sufficient time or not, and from this the grade of binocular vision can be determined.

Questions:

1. What do you mean by squint?
2. How is it detected?
3. What are the exercises prescribed for the correctment of squint?
4. What are the three stages of formation of binocular vision?

TONOMETRY

Tonometry is the technique by which the tension of the outer coat of the eye is assessed by measuring its impressibility.

Methods

(1) Digital Tonometry; and (2) Instrumental Tonometry.

Digital Tonometry

Normally Shiotz tonometer is used. To avoid cross infection the tonometer is well sterilized with ether or alcohol the agents are allowed to evaporate and then the tonometer is dipped in distilled water. If heat sterilized it is allowed to cool.

The instrument is placed on the test block or artificial cornea. The instrument must now read zero. Patient is placed on a couch or on a reclining chair and after the eye has been suitably anesthesised (1% Amethocaine) he is told to look upwards, preferably at a target spot on the ceiling. The surgeon holds the patient's eyelids apart, taking care not to press on the globe and holding the tonometer by its two side arms, sets it vertically upon the center of cornea. The cuff attached to the side arms supporting the instrument is now allowed to slide down the central cylinder so that the weight of the tonometer is taken by the eye and when the pressure is seen to be satisfactorily recorded by the lever, the reading is taken. First taken with 5.5 gms and then with 7.2 gms. The deflections of the pointer in each case on the scale are noted and from the calibrations provided with the instrument the tension can be directly read out. Normal tension of the eye is between 15-20 mm Hg.

Questions:

1. What is the normal tension of the eye?
2. In which conditions would you perform tonometry?

TESTS OF COLOUR VISION

The human eye can recognise about 150 different colours in the visible spectrum (400-750 μm) and can therefore detect differences of less than 3 m in wavelength. It is probable that three colours–red, green and blue are primary in that any other colour can be obtained by mixing these fundamental colours. The Young-Helmholtz theory suggests that there are three types of cones each perhaps possessing its own characteristic photosensitive substance, one type responding to red, another to green and yet another to blue light. The different colour sensations are supposed to be produced by stimulation of various combinations of these types of receptors. When the three cone types are stimulated equally a sensation of white light is produced.

The most common anomalies of colour vision are various types red, green weaknesses, inherited as sexlinked recessive condition, which occur in about 8% of males and 0.5% females. People with blue-green deficiency and with total colour blindness are rare.

Defects in Colour Vision are Tested By

1. **Holmgren's Skeins:** The subject is given a piece of wool and asked to match it by selection from an assortment of skeins of wool of various colours.
2. **Ishiara Charts:** These are printed with figures or designs in coloured circles on a background of circles to look similar, to a colour blind, to those of the figure. Colour blind people identify figures in pages of the chart, in which a normal person cannot read any letters or make out any pattern.
3. **The Edridge Green Lantern:** In which subject has to identify the colour of small illuminated area, the size of which can be varied. The device is used by board of trade to test would be engine drivers etc. for evidence of colour defective vision.

RETINOSCOPY

AIM

To assess the refractory state of the eye.

Requisites

Homatropine (2%), retinoscope.

Retinoscope

Retinoscopes is of two types:
1. Self illuminated.
2. Retinoscope where external source of light is used.

Procedure

Examiner sits at distance of 1arm/1 metre from the subject/ patient. Direct the subject to gaze at examiner's forehead.

By using plane mirror reflect the light into subject's pupil. Source of light is either from within the retinoscope while using self-illuminated retinoscope or external source that is behind the head of patient.

Light is reflected from the eye. See through the circular slit (in the retinoscope's centre). A "Red Glow" will be observed surrounded by a black shadow. This is called "RED REFLEX".

Now tilt the mirror of retinoscope horizontally and observe the movement of image/shadow of fundus. Image will move in same direction of tilting or against the tilting.

Hypermetropia: Image/shadow moves in same direction of tilting.

Myopia (>1D): Image will move in opposite direction.

Myopia (< -1D): Very faint shadow moving in same direction.

Emmetropia: Point to be noted is if the examiner is 1meter away from the subject, the combination of the subject's eye and the examiner's eye is equal to 1 Dioptre of myopia.

Uses

1. Objective and most practical method for estimating the condition of refraction.
2. **Astigmatism:** By performing retinoscopy in different meridians.
3. Malignering.
4. Illiterate subjects.
5. Infants.

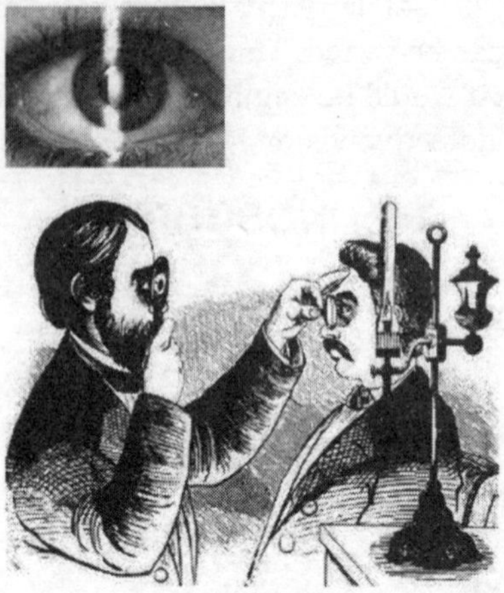

Fig. 26.2

Precautions

1. Retinoscopy is a dark room procedure. So should be conducted in dark room.
2. 1 metre distance to be maintained between examiner and subject.
3. Spectacles of subject should be removed before retinoscopy.

For better results CYCLOPLEGICS (Paralysis of ciliary muscles causing dilatation of pupil) must be used.

Questions:

1. What is the use of performing retinoscopy?
2. Why is a distance of one metre kept between examiner and patient?

27 TESTS OF VISUAL ACUITY

AIM

To assess the visual acuity of a subject.

Requisites

Snellen's charts for distant vision and Jaeger's test type for near vision.

Principle

Visual Acuity is defined as the reciprocal of the angle subtended at the nodal point, by two points which are separated by a distance and still distinguished as separate.

Visual acuity is different from visual threshold. **Visual threshold** is the minimum amount of light that can elicit a sensation of light.

A minimum of, at least 1minute angle should be subtended at the nodal point by the two distinct points, and based on this charts have been made, to test both, distant and near vision. These charts contain rows of letters of diminishing sizes. The person is asked to read these letters from a fixed distance. The size of the letter and the distance from which the subject is able to recognise it are noted and from this the visual acuity is determined.

PROCEDURE

Testing For Distant Vision: Using the Snellen's chart.

The **Snellen's chart** consists of 9 rows of letters printed in black. These are of decreasing sizes. The largest letter is placed at the top and the smallest at the bottom. The width of the lines forming the letters of the top row subtends an angle of one minute at the nodal point when viewed from a distance of 60 meters. This is marked as 60, at the side of the row. Similarly, the succeeding rows subtend an angle of 1 minute, when viewed from distances of 36 m, 24 m, 18 m, 12 m, 9 m, 6 m, 5 m (and are marked with the appropriate number at the side) i.e. 2nd row at a distance of 36 m, 3rd row at 24 m, 4th row at 18 m etc. Testing is done in daylight brightness or under artificial illumination with 100 foot candles brightness.

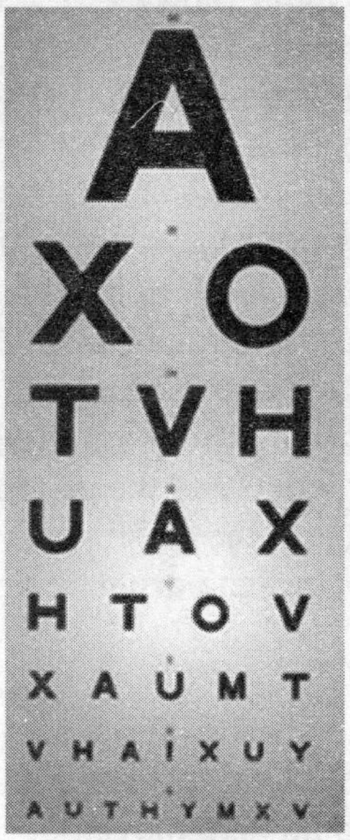

Fig. 27.1

Visual acuity (V) is recorded according to the formula V =d/D, where d is the distance at which the letters are read, and D that at which they should be read.

The patient is normally placed at a distance of 6 meters from the chart (d=6) and each eye is tested separately. The patient reads down the chart as far as he can.

A normal person should read upto the row marked as 6 (i.e. 7th row) with each eye. It shows that letters of this row are subtending an angle of 1 minute at a distance of 6 meters. In other words, the visual acuity is normal. It is expressed as 6/6. The numerator indicating the last row, which the subject is able to read (marked 6). If the subject is able to read only the first line (marked as 60) at a distance of 6 m then the visual acuity is expressed as 6/60.

If the subject is not able to read even the first row of letters from the distance of 6 meters, reduce the distance to 5 meters and assess the visual acuity. Now if he reads only the first row and not beyond that, the visual acuity is 5/60.

If the subject is not able to read even the first row of letters within a distance of 1 meter, i.e. his visual acuity is less than 1/60, **counting finger (CF) test** is done. Ask him to count your fingers at a distance of less than one meter. If he is able to count them at say ½ meter from his eye, it is expressed as CF at ½ meter.

In severe case, the subject may not be able to count the fingers even when the fingers are held closer to the eyes. In these cases, the subjects are asked to identify **hand movements (HM)**. Then it is expressed as HM at X cm.

In still severe cases, look for the perception of light (PL). The subject is taken to the dark room and light is shone into each eye separately. Observe if he is able to perceive light or not. It is expressed "Perception of light" (PL) or "No perception of light" (no PL). The light is then shown from all four quadrants–superior, inferior, nasal and temporal. This is called **projection of light (PR)**. If he is able to perceive the light, PR is + ve otherwise PR is –ve for that quadrant.

In some charts used for visual acuity figures such as broken circle or Landolt's C or Snellen's prong E, painted in black on white background in different sizes and in different positions are also used instead of different letters. These are used for small children and illiterates. The width of these figures or letters and the gap in them also subtend an angle of 1 minute at the nodal point when various sizes of them are kept at definite distance from the eye.

Precautions

1. Testing is done in good illumination.
2. Each eye should be tested separately.
3. Spectacles should be removed.
4. Any opacities in cornea should be excluded.

Testing for Near Vision

Jaeger's test type is used. This contains test types of progressively varying sizes, the notation being based on the printers "point" system. The smallest print is N 5. Here both eyes are tested together. The card is held at the normal reading distance. The near vision is recorded as the smallest type which the patient can read comfortably. Ability to read N6 is considered normal. Snellen's charts of different letters are also available, but now days are not used.

For illiterates near vision testing is done by similar charts as for distance vision i.e. Snellen's E or Landolt's C charts. Dots and square chart are also available. The subject counts the number of squares or circles (Fig. 26.2).

DISCUSSION

Various factors influencing visual acuity are as follows:

1. Retinal factors.
2. Optical factors.
3. Stimulus factors.

No. 7
1.50M
able treaty, the restitution of the standards and prisoners which had been taken in the defeat of Crassus. His generals, in the early part of his reign, attempted the reduction of Ethiopia and Arabia Felix. They marched near a thou-

No. 8
1.75M
sand miles to the south of the tropic; but the heat of the climate soon repelled the invaders, and protected the unwarlike natives of those sequestered regions

No. 9
2.00M
The northern countries of Europe scarcely deserved the expense and labor of conquest. The forests and morasses of Germany were

No. 10
2.25M
filled with a hardy race of barbarians who despised life when it was separated from freedom; and though, on the first

No. 11
2.50M
attack, they seemed to yield to the weight of the Roman power, they soon, by a signal

Fig. 27.2

Retinal Factors

Visual acuity is maximum at fovea centralis, where the cones are closely packed and each has a connection with a single ganglion cell. The periphery of the retina has the visual acuity of less than 1/30th of that of fovea. Foreign bodies in the eye, such as occur in industrial factories are more often found in the periphery of cornea than in the center, the flying object perceived much less easily at the periphery of the field of vision. Retinal diseases such as retinitis also decrease the acuity of vision.

Optical Factors

Errors of the refractive powers of the eye play an important part. Thus chromatic aberration leads to the reduction of visual acuity, whereas the use of nonchromatic light increases the visual acuity. Spherical aberration is decreased by pupillary constructions. Astigmatism, myopia and hypermetropia are the usual causes of low visual acuity.

Stimulus Factors

These are:

1. The intensity of stimulus.
2. Brightness contrast.
3. Duration of stimulus.

Viva-Voce Questions:

1. Comment on the visual acuity of the subject.
2. What is myopia, hypermetropia and astigmatism? How are they corrected?
3. What is night blindness?

28 EXAMINATION OF CRANIAL NERVES

AIM

To test the integrity of the cranial nerves.

Requisites

Tincture asafoetida, oil of cloves, oil of peppermint, sugar, salt, torch, tuning fork, Snellen's chart, Jaegger's chart, Ishiara chart, perimeter, cotton, fine needle, guaze, tubes with hot and cold water.

There are twelve pairs of cranial nerves in human beings, supplying sensory and motor fibers to the head, neck, thorax and abdomen. They serve a wide variety of functions, the examination of which leads to the knowledge of the functional state of these cranial nerves.

PROCEDURE

I. Olfactory Nerve

This subserves olfaction.

Each nostril is tested separately. Place some smelling substances like oil of cloves, oil of peppermint or tincture asafoetida in front of the nostril and ask the patient whether he can identify the smell. In testing the sense of smell, substances like ammonia should be avoided, as they irritate the fifth cranial nerve. Care is taken to exclude the local changes in the nostril itself before confirming that the nerve is at fault.

II. Optic Nerve

Subserves vision in all its faculties like light sense, form sense and colour sense.

Testing this nerve involves:

1. Tests for visual acuity.
2. Tests for field of vision.
3. Tests for colour vision.

III, IV and VI: Oculomotor, Trochlear and Abducent Nerves

These three nerves and their central connections are usually considered together and thus customarily tested together since they function as a physiological unit in the control of ocular movement.

The oculomotor nerve supplies all the extrinsic muscles of the eyeball except the superior oblique and the lateral rectus. It also supplies the levator palpabrae superioris and conveys parasympathetic fibers to the sphincter pupillae and ciliary muscle. The trochlear nerve supplies the superior oblique muscle and the abducent nerve supplies the lateral rectus.

The tests for these nerves include testing for:

1. Ocular movements;
2. Pupillary light reflex; and
3. Accommodation reflex.

Test for Ocular Movement

Test each eye separately. Fix the head of the subject with your hand. Ask him to follow your finger with his eye in various directions (up, down, left, right, diagonal and circular–clockwise and anti-clockwise). Assess if the movement is defective in any particular direction. (Recti act as elevators and depressors alone when the eye is in abduction and oblique act similarly in adduction. Testing movements of elevation and depression in both full abduction and adduction can easily assess their functions).

The action of levator palpabrae superioris is tested by fixing first the frontal belly of occipito-frontalis firmly with hand and asking the subject to look upwards. This can assess ptosis or drooping of the eyelids. If the frontal belly of occipito-frontalis is not fixed, it can obscure the impairment.

Examination of Pupil

a. Note the **size and shape:** Normally the pupil is circular.
b. **Pupillary Light Reflex:**
   Both direct and consensual light reflexes are tested. Throw a beam of light on one eye, shielding the other eye from the light. Direct light reflex causes constriction of the ipsilateral pupil while consensual light reflex causes constriction of contralateral pupil.

Direct Light Reflex

Examine each eye separately with the patient in a shady, indirectly illuminated place. Ask him to look into the distance, e.g. across the room, to be sure his accommodation is relaxed.

While constantly observing the subject's pupil, bring a bright light forwards from the side of his head and shine it directly into the eye to be tested. The pupil should contract almost immediately, then dilate again a little, and after undergoing a few slight oscillations, settle down to a smaller size. When the light is switched off the pupil will rapidly dilate to its previous diameter.

Consensual Light Reflex

It should be tested by keeping one eye in the shade while shining a bright light into the other. The effect on the pupil of the unilluminated eye is then observed. It is also seen to constrict.

c. **Accommodation Reflex**

Place your finger in front of the nose of the subject. Ask him to look at a distant object first and then suddenly to look at the finger. Look for the accommodation reflex, viz. convergence of the eyeballs and constriction of the pupil.

V. Trigeminal Nerve

It is sensory to the skin of scalp as far as the vertex, eyelids, skin of nose and ear and cheeks up to the angle of the mandible, the lips, teeth and lower part of face. Also supplies sensory mucous membranes of the nose, the roof of the mouth, part of the soft palate, the tonsils, the tongue, and eye: conjunctiva and cornea. It is motor to the muscles of mastication like temporalis and pterygoid muscle.

Tests for Sensory Function: Test the tactile sensations and temperature sensations in the usual manner in the areas of the face supplied by the nerve.

Tests for Corneal Reflex: Twist a wisp of cotton into a fine hair and lightly touch it to the lateral edge of cornea at its conjunctival margin, having asked the subject to gaze into the distance or at the ceiling. If the reflex is present, the subject blinks. Compare the two sides. This reflex can sometimes be tested more easily by lightly blowing a puff of air into each cornea in turn.

Tests for Motor Functions: Ask the subject to open his mouth partially. In lesions of the motor fibers of trigeminal nerve, the jaw is pushed to the paralysed side by the lateral pterygoid of the healthy side. Ask the subject to clench his teeth. If the motor function is intact, masseter and temporalis muscles stand out with equal prominence on both sides.

VII. Facial Nerve

It carries the taste fibers from anterior two thirds of tongue and is motor to all the muscles of face and scalp (except– the levator palpabrae superioris), the stapedius and platysma.

Inspection

In paralysis of facial nerve, the subject complains of dribbling of fluid while drinking, collection of food in the mouth on the paralysed side, obliteration of the nasolabial folds, loss of facial expression, drooping of the eyebrow or furrows of the eyebrow smoothed out, the eye is more widely open than on the normal side, and when the patient smiles the mouth is drawn toward the normal side. Note if these are present.

Test for Gustatory Function (Taste)

Hold the tip of the tongue with a gauze piece, dry the tongue with cotton, apply concentrated solution of sugar and ask the subject to write on a paper the sensation felt and its intensity and pleasantness. Then wash the tongue with water and dry it once again. Test in similar way solutions of common salt, citric acid and quinine.

Test for Motor Functions

1. Ask the subject to whistle. If there is paralysis of the facial nerve, the subject will not be able to do this.
2. Ask him to blow his cheeks after inflating his mouth with air. Tap the cheeks. If facial nerve is involved there is muscle weakness and air escapes out of the mouth.
3. Ask the subject to shut his eyes tightly. He will not be able to close the eye completely on the affected side. Try to open the eyes while he attempts to keep them closed. It is difficult to open the eyes in normal persons when tightly closed, but in facial nerve paralysis, it can be opened very easily.
4. Ask the subject to smile or show his upper teeth. If there is unilateral facial paralysis, the mouth is drawn to the healthy side.
5. Paralysis of stapedius may cause hyperacusis (low tones are perceived loudly). Note if this is the case.

VIII. Vestibulo-cochlear Nerve

The vestibular component of this nerve subserves vestibular function i.e. in equilibrium and the cochlear component subserves audition (hearing).

Tests for Vestibular Function

In lesions, patients normally complain of **vertigo,** usually describing it as giddiness or dizziness. **Nystagmus** i.e. involuntary rhythmic to and fro movement of the eye ball may also be observed. Specialised tests like **rotational tests, calorie tests** etc. are available for testing this component of nerve.

Tests for Cochlear Function

If the cochlear part of the nerve is affected there is deafness. It can be assessed by the following tests:

Voice Test

Each ear is tested separately. Find out the distance at which the patient can hear the whispered or the spoken words. Compare this with the normal.

Watch Test

Each ear is tested separately. Ask the subject to close his eyes. Bring a ticking watch towards the ear of the patient, which is initially held beyond the range of hearing. When the patient says that he can hear the ticking of the watch, note the distance and compare with the normal. In both the above tests, when one ear is tested, the other is plugged with cotton.

Tuning Fork Tests

These tests are used to differentiate the type of deafness: conduction deafness or nerve deafness. These tests are performed using a tuning fork vibrating at 250 or 512 Hz (cps). The observer must set the tuning fork into vibration by striking the prongs against a hard surface, making sure it is vibrating by listening to the vibrations and only then using it on the subject.

a. **Rinne's Test:** Each ear is tested separately for its ability to hear both through the bone (bone conduction) and through the air (air conduction). Place the base of a vibrating tuning fork on the mastoid process of the subject and when he indicates that he can no longer hear the sound, hold the tuning fork in air next to the ear. If the hearing is normal, the subject can still hear the sound for about 45 seconds more than the bone conduction (Rinne's test is positive). In conduction deafness, the subject does not hear vibrations in air conduction after the bone conduction is over. (Rinne's test is negative). In total or complete nerve deafness, no sound is heard either by way of air or bone conduction.
b. **Weber's Test:** In this, only bone conduction is tested in both the ears simultaneously. Place the base of the vibrating tuning fork on the vertex of the skull. If hearing is normal the sound is heard equally on both sides. In conduction deafness, the sound is lateralised to the diseased ear, i.e. the sound is louder in the diseased ear, because the masking effect of the environmental noise is absent on the diseased side. In nerve deafness, the sound is lateralised to the normal ear.
c. **Schwabach's Test:** The bone conduction of the subject is compared to that of a normai subject. In conduction deafness, bone conduction is longer in patients due to exclusion of masking effect of the environmental noise. In nerve deafness, bone conduction is shorter in patients.

Audiometry

Audiometry is of two types:

(a) Pure tone audiometry (subjective test).
(b) Brainstem evoked response audiometry (BERA) which is objective.

These audiometric tests are performed in ENT or electrophysiology labs. In pure tone audiometry, subject is tested for hearing as different pure tones, whereas in BERA functional integrity of the brainstem auditory pathway is tested by auditory evoked responses *(For details See Chapter 36–Evoked Potentials)*. The latter test can be used in newborn, infants and young non-cooperative children. BERA can also be used for diagnosing brainstem lesions, tumours, demyelinating diseases.

IX. Glossopharyngeal Nerve

It subserves **taste functions** from the posterior one third of the tongue. Tested in the usual way.

It is **motor** to middle pharyngeal constrictor. It subserves reflex functions like **palatine and pharyngeal reflexes.** Tickle the back of the pharynx and note if reflex contraction occurs.

X. Vagus Nerve

It is sensory and motor to heart, lungs and abdominal viscera, and motor to palate, pharynx and larynx.

Patients with vagus paralysis complain of **regurgitation of fluid** through the nose while swallowing.

Palatine reflex is absent.

Direct Examination of the Soft Palate

Place the patient facing the light with his mouth open and introduce a tongue depressor. Ask the subject to say "Ah". Watch the movement of both arches of soft palate. Normally they move equally on both sides with the uvula (median raphe) remaining in the midline. If there is unilateral vagus nerve paralysis, there is no movement of palate on that side and the median raphe will be pulled towards the healthy side. In bilateral paralysis the whole of the soft palate remains motionless.

XI. Accessory Nerve

This is entirely motor and supplies the trapezoid and sternocleidomastoid muscles.

To test the integrity of this nerve, ask the patient to **shrug his shoulders against resistance**.

To test the sternocleidomastoid muscle, offer resistance on one side and ask him to **rotate the chin** towards the opposite side.

XII. Hypoglossal Nerve

It is purely motor to the musculature of the tongue.

Ask the subject to **protrude the tongue** as far as possible. See whether it lies in the center or deviates to one side. In normal individuals, it lies in the center. In hypoglossal nerve paralysis, it deviates to the paralysed side.

Ask the subject to perform various movements like **moving the tongue** from side to side, licking the cheeks with it etc. Look for fasciculation's and wasting of the tongue. Presence of these indicates a paralysis of hypoglossal nerve.

29

HISTORY TAKING AND GENERAL EXAMINATION

The objective of history taking is to get information about the patient's present illness, past illness, personal habits and family history, all for the purpose of diagnosis.

Regarding the present illness, it gives useful data to the system involved, the intensity, progress or regression of the disease, all being important for diagnosis. In some cases, history may be the only pointer to the disease e.g. angina pectoris (pain in the chest) may be the only evidence of ischaemic heart disease in absence of all other clinical or laboratory investigations.

The following scheme is usually employed in recording of the history:

1. Name:
2. Age:
3. Sex: if F, menstrual onset/cessation
4. Race: Profession
5. Marital status and children if any:
6. Residential address:

This is followed by:

1. History of the present illness.
2. History of the past illness.
3. Personal history.
4. Family history.

It is emphasized that the plan cannot always be rigidly employed. In an unconscious patient history may not be obtained from the patient. In critically ill patient, the history must be short and in a medical emergency the treatment should begin even before the history.

History of the Present Illness

History of the present illness is recorded under two headings:

(i) Patient's presenting or chief complaints.
(ii) Onset, duration and progress of the complaints.

Each of the complaint is then elaborated regarding its onset, duration and progress. This information should include whether the symptoms were rapid or gradual in onset, whether the duration of the illness is short or prolonged and whether each of the symptoms is progressing, stationary or regressing. Most of this account should come spontaneously from the patient, the physician merely guiding the narration whenever necessary. By this time a fair outline of the disease should be obvious. An enquiry should be made about other diagnostically important symptoms that the patient might have forgotten to mention. Some time such an enquiry reveals that the symptoms started earlier than the patient thought and apparently recent illness may actually be an old ailment. Finally, if the treatment is taken for the present illness its effectiveness must be recorded.

History of the present illness recorded in the manner mentioned above should cover all the symptoms and their progress and yet it should be brief. However, practice and skill is required to prepare concise account. Some patients can narrate the history precisely, others keep on presenting irrelevant data into which the main symptoms tend to get lost. In these patients to make the history brief and precise, one may resort to asking "leading" questions which suggest the answer themselves. In general leading questions should be avoided. Properly recorded history of the present illness usually makes the diagnosis obvious.

History of Past Illness

History of past illness either recent or remote may have a bearing on the diagnosis of the present illness. For example, in a patient with valvular heart disease, history of rheumatic fever in childhood points to the cause of the disease. History of past illness should be recorded under the following headings:

1. History of illness similar to the present condition.
2. History of all major illnesses.
3. History of operations in the past.
4. History of venereal disease when relevant.
5. History of allergic reaction to certain drugs.
6. In children, history of infectious diseases and vaccinations together with their last booster doses.
7. Mode of delivery in children, e.g. by forceps when relevant.

Personal History

Recording of the personal history like appetite, bowel movements, habits or occupation may provide a pointer to the diagnosis. For example, recent loss of appetite in the elderly may point to stomach cancer, smoking predisposes to lung cancer or ischaemic heart disease; occupation in asbestos industry predisposes to tuberculosis of the lungs. Following points should be included in the personal history:

1. Appetite.
2. Diet.
3. Bowel habits.
4. Sleep.
5. Micturition history.
6. Menstrual history in women.
7. Habits of smoking, tobacco chewing, alcohol intake, excessive tea or coffee.
8. Occupation.
9. Socio-economic status.

Family History

Family history provides information of diagnostic importance in infectious disease and hereditary disorders. As an example, in children with fever and skin rash, history of measles or other exanthematous fever points to that diagnosis. Family history also informs about overcrowding, sanitary conditions and socio-economic status. This may be useful in the diagnosis as well as planning the treatment. The following should be recorded in the family history:

1. History of the illness that is same or similar to that of the patient.
2. History of hereditary disorders likes diabetes mellitus, hemophilia, and high blood pressure.
3. History of infectious diseases.
4. Histories of allergic disorders like asthma, eczema etc.
5. History of sudden deaths in the family members when relevant.
6. Socio-economic conditions, overcrowding and disorders of malnutrition in the family.

GENERAL EXAMINATION

General examination involves observation of the patient from head to foot for features of diagnostic help. It is usually carried out under the following headings, each of which may provide useful information:

1. **Decubitus:** This term implies position adopted by the patient in bed. For example orthopneic decubitus in cardiac failure, ophisthotonus of tetanus etc.
2. **Mental State:** Mental state is examined for patient's orientation in time, space and person, his emotional state, and his abnormalities of behavior. These features are usually obvious during history taking. Examples are delirium in fever, psychiatric manifestations of neurosyphilis.
3. **Temperature, Pulse and Respiration (TPR):** These findings are altered in many conditions. TPR chart is maintained in all patients for monitoring the progress of the disease. In addition, the pattern of temperature is diagnostic in conditions like malaria whereas rate and rhythm of respiration and pulse characterize some chest and cardiac disorders.
4. **Built:** Built is judged from the height, weight and chest girth. According to the built, subjects are considered average, esthetic (short and stalky) or asthenic (tall and thin).
5. **Nutrition:** To examine nutrition one looks for evidence of undernutrition or overnutrition (obesity). Both predispose to certain disease. Undernutrition may be characterized by (a) loss of weight due to poor caloric intake, (b) manifestations of a vitaminosis as scurvy (vit. C deficiency) or pellagra (vit. B deficiency) (c) anemia due to poor iron intake. Deficit water intake leads to dehydration. Deficit of protein intake leads to wasting of muscles and edema.
6. **Head:** The head should be examined for size and shape. Small head (microcephaly) is usually observed in mentally retarded person. Large head (hydrocephalus) occurs when there is obstruction to circulation of cerebrospinal fluid. In children, increase in the girth of the head according to the age is a useful guide to the development of brain.
7. **Face:** Face should be observed for general appearance or "Facies" that characterize some conditions. For example, exophthalmic goiter, myxoedema, myasthenia gravis etc.
8. **Eyes:**
   (i) **Conjunctiva** should be examined for:
      a. PALLOR due to anemia.
      b. CYANOSIS (bluish discoloration) which occurs in congenital hearts disease or respiratory disease.
      c. DRYNESS that indicates dehydration.
   (ii) The **sclera** should be examined for:
      a. Yellowish pigmentation indicating jaundice.
      b. Evidence of hemorrhages indicating scurvy or a bleeding disorder.
   (iii) The **cornea** should be examined for xerophthalmia (sign of vit. A deficiency).
   (iv) The state of **pupils** (constricted or dilated) provides useful information.
9. **Mouth:** Mouth should be examined for:
   - **Breath:** e.g. Odour of acetone indicates diabetic acidosis. Bad odour may be due to pyorrhea (Halitosis).
   - **Lips:** Pallor indicates anemia and bluish discoloration indicates cyanosis.
   - **Gums:** Bleeding tendency indicates scurvy or gingivitis. Blueline at the margins suggests lead poisoning.

- **Tongue:** (a) Pallor suggests anemia, (b) Cyanosis occurs in congenital heart disease, (c) Dryness indicates dehydration, (d) Red, angry-looking tongue indicates glossitis due to vit. B deficiency, (e) Presence of ulceration suggests aphthous ulcers or cancer, particularly at the base of the tongue.
- **Buccal cavity:** Ulcer due to cancer is common in our country due to habit of chewing tobacco or pan.
- **Tonsils:** Recent enlargement indicates tonsillitis. Presence of membrane may be due to tonsillitis or diphtheria.

10. **Neck:** Neck should be examined for enlarge thyroid gland or lymphadenopathy engorgement of the neck veins.
11. **Lymph Nodes:** Lymph nodes should be examined for their enlargement in the neck, axilla, supratrochlear region and groins. Common causes of lymphadenopathy are tuberculosis, infection or cancer in area drained and lymphomas.
12. **Nails:** The nails should be examined for: (a) Pallor, (b) Cyanosis, (c) Abnormalities of shape-concave spoon-shaped nail (Koilonychia) indicates iron deficiency anemia.
13. **Fingers:** Fingers should be examined for clubbing. It is characterized by obliteration of the angle between the base of the nail and the adjacent skin. It occurs in congenital cyanotic heart disease and respiratory disease.
14. **Skin:** Skin should be examined for:
    - i. Pallor indicating - Anemia.
    - ii. Bluish discoloration - Cyanosis.
    - iii. Yellow discoloration - Jaundice.
    - iv. Abnormal pigmentation.
    - v. Evidence of vitamin deficiency such as pellagra, scurvy or phrenoderma.
    - vi. Skin eruptions, e.g. those occurring in exanthematous fevers like measles, smallpox etc.
    - vii. State of hydration and texture. Wrinkled, inelastic skin occurring in dehydration due to fluid loss. Dry course skin in myxoedema.
    - viii. Hair loss, e.g., male pattern baldness or abnormal hair growth in women (hirsutism).
15. **Oedema:** Edema of subcutaneous tissues is characterized by "pitting" on pressure. Edema occurs initially in dependent parts (ankles or sacrum) in congestive cardiac failure, hypoproteinaemia, liver disease etc.
16. **Bones and Joints:** Bones and joints should be examined for swelling and deformities, e.g., kyphosis, scoliosis etc.

Observation Table

Name
Age
Sex
Marital Status
Race
Address
History of Present Illness
    Chief Complaints:
    Relevant History:
Relevant Past History
Relevant Personal History
Relevant Family History

GENERAL EXAMINATION

- Decubitus
- Mental State
- Vital Sign
    - Temperature
    - Pulse Rate
    - Blood Pressure
    - Respiratory Rate
- Built
- Nutritional Status
- Head
- Face/Facies
- Eyes
- Conjunctiva
    - Pallor
    - Cyanosis
- Sclera
    - Icterus
    - Evidence of hemorrhage
- Cornea
- Mouth
    - Breath
    - Lips
    - Gums
    - Tongue
    - Buccal cavity
    - Tonsils
- Neck
- Lymph Nodes
- Nails
- Fingers for Clubbing
- Skin
- Oedema
- Bones and Joints

30

CLINICAL EXAMINATION OF CARDIOVASCULAR SYSTEM, RESPIRATORY SYSTEM

CARDIOVASCULAR SYSTEM

AIM

To perform clinical examination of cardiovascular system.

REQUISITES

Stethoscope, measuring tape, and sphygmomanometer.

PROCEDURE

The examination is done in the following order:

1. **History of the Patient:** The present complaint, history of present illness, menstrual history, treatment history, family history, etc. are noted. These recordings help in getting an accurate account of the subject's complaint and in seeing this against the background of his life as a whole.
2. **Examination of the Subject:** First the examination of the general state of the patient is done: the general appearance of illness, mental state of the patient, his expression, build, state of nutrition, skin colour, body hair, limb examination etc. are done under this.
   1. Examination of cardiovascular system is done under the following headings: (1) General Examination and (2) Systemic Examination.

GENERAL EXAMINATION

Look for:

1. **Pallor:** In lower palpebral conjunctiva, **nails and** mucous membrane.
2. **Cyanosis:** Bluish or purplish tint in lips, nails **and** tip of nose.
3. **Clubbing:** In the fingers, characterised by obliteration of the angle between the base of the nail and adjacent skin.
4. **Edema:** On medial malleolus, shin of tibia and sacrum.
5. **Vital Signs:** (i) Pulse (ii) B.P. (iii) Respiration rate (iv) Temperature.

A. Examination of the Pulse

It is always better to feel all the peripheral pulses, but usually radial pulse is the one, which is always felt. It is best felt with the tips of the fingers, the subject's forearm being pronated and slightly flexed. Patient must be fully relaxed before the examination. The following observations should be made:

i. **Rate of Pulse:** Pulse is counted for 1 min. Pulse rate (PR) varies with age: PR = 60-100/min in adults and 130-140/min in newborn. Slow pulse is called bradycardia and fast pulse tachycardia. Pulse rate is increased during exercise, anxiety, fever, and thyrotoxicosis and decreased in myxoedema, typhoid and incomplete heart blocks.

ii. **Rhythm of Pulse:** Normally the pulse is regular i.e. it beats at a regular interval. Irregular pulse is called arrhythmia. Sinus arrhythmia is increased rate of pulse during inspiration and decreased rate of pulse during expiration. It is a physiological phenomenon caused by change in vagal tone. Irregular rhythm is seen in atrial fibrillation and due to extrasystoles.

iii. **Character of Pulse:** This is most satisfactorily done by palpating a large vessel. Character of pulse takes into account the volume of pulse, its force and tension.

iv. **Volume of Pulse:** By this is meant the amplitude of movement of vessel wall during the passage of the pulse wave. The volume of equivalent pulses on two sides should be compared.

v. **Condition of Vessel Wall:** Sufficient pressure should be exerted on the brachial artery to abolish pulsation in the radial artery which should be then rolled beneath the fingers against the underlying bones. In young persons, arteries cannot be felt. But in old people they are easily palpable.

vi. **Radial-Femoral Delay:** This is examined in the femoral pulses in comparison with the radial by simultaneous examination of the two pulses. The presence or absence, or delay in the femoral pulses in comparison with the radial is noted.

B. Blood Pressure

Blood pressure of the person is taken in sitting and standing posture.

SYSTEMIC EXAMINATION

Subject should be in lying down posture and examiner on the right side of the subject.

Inspection and Palpation

Patient should be examined in a good light, at an angle of 45° if possible. Note the following points:

i. Shape of chest and precordium.
ii. Neck veins.
iii. Cardiac impulse.
iv. Veins on chest wall.
v. Other pulsations.
vi. Position of trachea.
vii. Thrills.

Shape of Chest and Precordium: The chest wall is exposed well, while the patient lies supine or sits if orthopneic. The precordium, which is the area of the chest wall overlying the heart, is observed tangentially (from foot end of the patient or from the side) for the following points:

- Bulging or depression.
- Presence of dilated or engorged veins.

Neck Veins: They communicate directly with the right atrium. Changes in the mean pressure within them, together with pulsation that occurs with each cardiac cycle give direct information about the mean pressure changes in the right atrium during cardiac cycle.

The neck veins should be examined when the patient is reclining at an angle of 45°. They normally show slight pulsation and two or three small waves can be distinguished in each cardiac cycle. There is however, a mean level and the perpendicular height of level over the right atrium indicates the mean hydrostatic pressure in the right atrium. The manubrium sterni is a convenient reference point for measuring the right atrial pressure.

Cardiac Impulse: It refers to the character of the apex beat, other pulsations, palpable murmurs (thrills) and heart sounds.

Apex Beat: It is customary to locate the apex beat as the outermost and lower most point of definite cardiac pulsation. Normal position of apex beat is 3½" internal to the midclavicular line in the left 5th intercostal space. Normally the apex beat raises the palpating finger without an undue thrust.

- Apex beat is displaced in scoliosis, pleural effusion, pulmonary fibrosis, and in cardiac enlargement.
- Forceful thrust of apex beat felt in cardiac hypertrophy.
- Feeble diffuse impulse with the position changed towards axilla is felt in cardiac dilatation.
- Force is increased in nervous persons, after exercise and in hyperthyroidism.

Veins on Chest Wall are seen in:

1. Patients with transparent and thin skin.
2. When an intrathoracic growth or aneurysm obstructs the blood flow to heart.
3. Portal hypertension.

Position of Trachea: Feel for the trachea in the suprasternal notch and decide whether it is placed centrally or not. A significant displacement of trachea or cardiac impulse can occur in various disease conditions e.g. pneumothorax, pleural effusion, pulmonary kochs or bronchopneumonia.

Thrills: Any sound or murmur, which is loud enough to be palpable, is called a thrill. It transmits to the hand, a sensation like the purring of a cat.

Loud first sound in mitral stenosis is often palpable and sounds of aortic and pulmonary valve closure are also often palpable in systemic and pulmonary hypertensions respectively.

PERCUSSION
(Details in Respiratory System Examination)

By percussion an attempt is made to define the borders of the heart. By percussing in the 4th intercostal space from the left lung towards the heart, it is possible to define the left border. It is found about ½" internal to midclavicular line. Right border of the heart is just next to the right of sternum at the level of 4th rib; cardiac dullness is increased in pericardial effusion and aortic aneurysms. The upper border of the heart cannot be defined accurately as the dullness of the heart tissue continues with the dullness of the big vessels. Similarly, the lower border of the heart cannot be defined as it lies in relation with the diaphragm and the left lobe of the liver below it.

AUSCULTATION

This is the listening to the heart with a stethoscope and it gives information concerning the function of heart valves and the state of myocardium and pericardium. There are four areas of auscultation:

i. *Mitral area:* At the apex of the heart.
ii. *Tricuspid area:* In left 4th I/C space just lateral to sternal border.
iii. *Aortic area:* At the junction of right 2nd costal cartilage with the sternum.
iv. *Pulmonary area:* In the left 2nd I/C space 2 cm lateral to the sternal border.

First Heart Sound

This is the onset of ventricle systole. Mitral and tricuspid valves close, almost simultaneously to give the first heart sound. It is soft and low-pitched. Duration is more than second heart sound. i.e. 0.15 sec. It is best heard at the mitral area.

Second Heart Sound

Closure of aortic and pulmonary valves gives rise to the two components of second heart sound. It is sharper; high-pitched, shorter than the first sound i.e. 0.12 sec. It is best heard at aortic and pulmonary areas.

PROFORMA (CVS EXAMINATION)

Name:
Age:
Sex:

I. Symptoms:

1. Dyspnoea
2. Pain in chest
3. Palpitation
4. Cyanosis
5. Edema
6. Syncope
7. Asthma

II. General Examination:

1. Build
2. Nourishment
3. Pallor in nails and conjunctiva
4. Lymph glands
5. Tongue

III. Examination of Heart:

1. Inspection:

A. Precordium
B. Pulsations
C. Apex beat
D. Neck veins

2. Palpation:

A. Apex beat
 Situation
 Character
 Thrill
B. Palpable pulsations of carotid in neck.
C. Radial pulse
D. B.P.

3. Percussion:

Cardiac borders
Left
Right
Upper
Lower

4. Auscultation:

Mitral area
Pulmonary area
Aortic area
Tricuspid area
Murmurs

RESPIRATORY SYSTEM

AIM

To examine the respiratory system of a given subject.

REQUISITES

Stethoscope, couch or examination table, measuring tape.

PROCEDURE

The examination is done in the following order:

1. **History of the Patient:**
 The present complaint, history of present illness, menstrual history, treatment history, family history, etc. are noted. These recordings help in getting an accurate account of the subject's complaint and in seeing this against the background of his life as a whole.
2. **Examination of the Subject:**
 a. **General examination:** It is done to determine the general state of the patient, the general appearance of illness, mental state of the patient, his expression, build, state of nutrition, skin colour, body hair, limb examinations etc.
 b. **Systemic examination:** The respiratory system is examined by examination of the chest in the following order:
 (i) Inspection, (ii) Palpation, (iii) Percussion, and (iv) Auscultation.

The patient should be sitting up or lying down and the examiner should be on the right side of the subject. The examination should be done in good light.

INSPECTION

Size and Shape of Chest: Normally the chest is bilaterally symmetrical and on cross-section is ellipsoidal, its transverse diameter being more than anteroposterior diameter (7:5). The sub-costal angle is about 90°, being more acute in males. The shape of the chest varies with the build of the individual. Size and shape get altered in different diseases e.g. pigeon chest in rickets and barrel shaped chest in emphysema.

Movements of the Chest: Movements are observed from the foot end of bed tangentially and the following points are noted:

i. **Rate of Respiration:** The rate of respiration for a normal adult is about 14-18/min, but upto 22 if the patient is nervous under examination. Tachypnoea or increased respiratory rate is an important sign of pulmonary diseases. To determine the rate of respiration, the hand is placed lightly on the chest or upper abdomen of the subject, and the movements of the chest are counted for a minute.

ii. **The Rhythm of Respiration:** Normally it is regular with inspiration longer than expiration. But if the patient is conscious of respiration, it becomes irregular. Hence this is to be observed when the patient is off his guard. If either inspiration or expiration is unduly prolonged, it is abnormal.

iii. **Type:** In males and some females the respiration is abdominothoracic but in majority of females it is thoracoabdominal in nature.

iv. **Movement:** Normally both sides of chest wall move uniformly and there is no bulging or indrawing of the intercostal spaces. Chest expansion can be measured with a tape around the chest at the level of nipples. In a fit young man it may be 5-8 cms.

v. **The Ratio between Respiration and Pulse:** In health this ratio is about 1:4.

PALPATION

1. First palpate any obvious swelling or where the patient complains of pain. Look at the face rather than the part under examination, so as to avoid causing unnecessary pain.
2. **Position of Cardiac Impulse and Trachea:** Feel for the trachea in the suprasternal notch and decide whether it is placed centrally or deviated to one or other side by its relation to the suprasternal notch and the insertion of the sternomastoids. Compare the prominence of clavicular head of sternocleidomastoid muscle on each side. Undue prominence on one side indicates tracheal shift to that side. The normal apex beat can be palpated at the fifth left intercostal space, half an inch internal to the midclavicular line.
3. **Nature of Respiratory Movements:** It is then studied to make certain that the two sides of the chest move to approximately the same extent. This is done by fixing the fingertips of either hand at the patient's sides and making the tips of the thumbs just meet in the middle line in front of the chest. The patient is directed to take a full inspiration, when the distance of departure of the thumbs from the middle line indicates the extent of expansion of either half of the chest.
4. **Tactile Vocal Fremitus:** The palm of the hand is applied flat on the chest. The patient is then told to repeat 'one, one, one' or 'ninety-nine' in a clear voice. Distinct vibrations can be detected during this and one must determine whether the vibrations in corresponding areas on the two sides of the chest are approximately equal in intensity. These vibrations perceived by examining hand are set up by the voice and are conducted from the larynx by the trachea and bronchi to the smaller tubes within the lungs and then through the lung tissue to the surface. This vocal fremitus is necessarily much diminished where the heart encroaches on the left lung. Vocal fremitus is increased in consolidation of the lung and diminished in pleural effusion.

Percussion and Auscultation

Entire chest to be examined making sure that the areas examined correspond exactly with each other on the two sides.

Position of Choice of the Patient

Sitting up but can be done in standing or lying down position. Face should be turned sideways to avoid breathing into the examiner.

For Examination:

- **Front side:** Sitting with head and shoulder erect.
- **Back side:** Sitting with subject bending forward with the head flexed and crossed arms resting on the shoulders.
- **Axillary region:** Sitting position with both arms on head.

It is done to determine the state of underlying lung tissue.

PERCUSSION

The middle finger of the left hand (pleximeter finger) is placed firmly on the part, which is to be percussed. The back of its middle phalanx is then struck with the tip of the middle finger of the right hand (percussing finger). The stroke should be delivered from the wrist and finger joints, not from the elbow, and the percussing finger should be so bent that when the blow is delivered, its terminal phalanx is at right angles to the metacarpal bones and strikes the pleximeter fingers perpendicularly. As soon as the blow has been given, the striking finger must be raised. The percussion is to be done from a more resonant area to a less resonant area. The pleximeter must be parallel to the edge of the organ percussed. A firm contact must be there between the pleximeter and the chest surface, there should not be any air space in between.

Beginning in front, the examiner should tap lightly and directly (without pleximeter finger) on the most prominent point of each clavicle being sure that the points examined correspond exactly with each other.

The patient's attitude must be comfortable and his arms and shoulders must be placed symmetrically. The observer should have two objects in mind: (i) first to make a comparison of the percussion note in comparable areas on the two sides and (ii) to map out the limits of lung resonance particularly at the apices, bases and the area of cardiac dullness.

The normal degree of resonance varies from individual to individual and in different parts of the chest in the same individual, being most resonant below the clavicles and scapulae where the muscles are relatively thin, and least resonant over the scapulae.

The lower limits of the lung: (i) Of the right lung: lies over the liver and is thin, the lower border is found to lie in the mammary line at the 6th rib, in the mid axillary line at the 8th rib and in the scapular line at the 10th rib. (ii) Of the left lung: overlaps the stomach, so the transition is from the lung resonance to the tympanitic resonance of the stomach. Posteriorly, there is dullness due to spleen and various other solid organs, and hence resembles the dullness of the right side. Lung resonance is impaired in consolidation, fibrosis of lung, thickened pleura, and pleural effusion. Resonance is increased in pneumothorax.

AUSCULTATION

Auscultation (listening with the stethoscope) must be performed all over the chest and the two sides should be compared. The patient should breath with his mouth open, regularly and deeply but not noisily. Three observations must be made at each point auscultated:

i. Character of the breath sounds;
ii. The character of the vocal resonance; and
iii. The presence or absence of other sounds.

i. Character of Breath Sounds: May be (a) Vesicular or (b) Bronchial.

a. Vesicular Sounds: Produced by passage of air in and out of normal lung tissue, and are heard all over the chest under normal conditions. Typically heard in axillary and infra-scapular regions. Characteristics of these sounds are: (i) the inspiratory sound is fairly intense and is audible during the whole of the act; (ii) the expiratory sound follows that of inspiration without a distinct pause. It only remains audible during the earlier part of the expiratory phase, and under the normal conditions the inspiratory sound is heard for at least twice as long as the expiratory. Vesicular breathing is low pitched and rustling in character.

b. Bronchial Sounds: Produced by the passage of air through the trachea and large bronchi. Under normal conditions they can be heard by listening over the trachea, but they are not heard over normal lung tissue. In disease, however, these sounds may be conducted from the bronchi to the chest wall. Characteristics of these sounds:

- The inspiratory sound is moderately intense. It becomes inaudible shortly before the end of inspiration. Its quality is harsh and aspirate.
- The expiratory sound is generally more intense than the inspiratory; the pitch is often higher, the duration extends through the greater part of expiration, being as long as, or even longer than, the inspiratory sound. In quality, resembles the inspiratory sound, being aspirate in character.
- There is a definite gap between inspiration and expiration.

ii. Character of Vocal Resonance: When the patient repeats the words 'one, one, one' or 'ninety-nine', the ear perceives, not the distinct syllables, but a resonant sound, the intensity of which depends on the loudness and depth of the patient's voice and on the conductivity of the lungs. It varies in intensity even in health being more intense the nearer the stethoscope is to the larger bronchi. Vocal resonance of normal intensity generally conveys the impression of being produced just at the chest-piece of the stethoscope. Vocal resonance is increased in consolidation and diminished in pleural thickening and effusion.

iii. Added Sounds: These may arise in the lung or in the pleura. Movement of the stethoscope on the patient's skin, or of the observer's hands or clothes against the stethoscope may produce sounds resembling pleural friction. Abnormal sounds in diseased states are:

a. Rhonchi: These are prolonged uninterrupted noises, arising in the bronchi and are due to partial obstruction of their lumen, by swelling of the mucosa, by viscid secretion or by constriction of bronchial smooth muscle, e.g., bronchial asthma.

b. Crepitations: These are discontinuous crackling or bubbling sounds which may be produced in the alveoli, the bronchi or the cavities. They sound like the bursting of air bubbles, and indicate the presence of fluid secretions. They may be fine or coarse. The opening up of collapsed alveoli probably causes fine crepitations. Can be imitated by rolling a few hairs between the finger and thumb in front of the ear. Coarse crepitations are bubbling or clicking noises which can probably arise in many sites, including large and small branches of the bronchial tree or in cavities, and may be heard at almost any phase of or during the whole of respiration, e.g., pulmonary oedema.

c. Pleural Rub or Friction Sounds: Seen in pleurisy at the stage when exudation is not abundant enough to separate the inflamed and roughened pleural surfaces. It has a creaking or rubbing character.

Questions:

1. What information is derived from testing the vocal fremitus of the subject?
2. Name the muscles involved in the process of:
   a. Normal inspiration.
   b. Deep inspiration.
3. What is abdominal and thoracic breathing?
4. What is a paradoxical breathing?

Clinical Examination of Respiratory System

Name:
Age:
Sex:

I. Symptoms:
1. Cough
2. Haemoptysis
3. Pain in chest
4. Dyspnoea
5. Fever

II. General Examination:
1. Body build
2. Nourishment
3. Cyanosis
4. Clubbing
5. Neck veins
6. Accessory muscles of respiration
7. Lymph nodes

III. Examination of Respiratory System:

A. Inspection:
1. Upper respiratory passage
2. Form of chest
3. Position of apex beat
4. Movements of chest
   a. Rate
   b. Rhythm
   c. Type
   d. Equality
   e. Respiration-Pulse ratio

B. Palpation
1. Chest diameter
2. Position of trachea
3. Position of apex beat
4. Movements of chest
5. Tactile vocal fremitus

C. Percussion–dull/resonant

D. Auscultation
1. Air entry
2. Breath sounds – Vesicular
   Bronchial
3. Vocal resonance
4. Abnormal sounds

31 EXAMINATION OF MOTOR AND SENSORY SYSTEM

EXAMINATION OF MOTOR SYSTEM

AIM

Examination of the motor system.

REQUIREMENTS

Percussion hammer, sharp object, measuring tape.

PROCEDURE

The motor system should be examined with the following aspects of motor functions in mind.

I. Bulk of Muscles

Most easily estimated by inspection and palpation e.g.: Take two similar points on the two arms and measure and compare the diameter. Then palpate the corresponding muscles and compare the feel of these muscles.

The muscles may be normal, smaller or larger than normal.

On palpation may they be flabby, soft or hard and inelastic.

II. Tone of Muscles

Is the state of tension due to inherent contraction found in healthy muscles. The degree of tone can be estimated by handling the limbs and moving them passively at their various joints.

Tone may be:

- Normal.
- Hypotonia as in spinal cord lesions or motor nerve lesion.
- Hypertonia as in upper motor neuron type lesions.

III. Strength of Muscles

Watch the patient walking, jumping, hopping, standing up from lying and sitting positions.

Weakness or paresis is often graded according to Medical Research Council Scale as Grade 0-5.

Grade 0 : Complete paralysis.

Grade 1 : A flicker of contraction only.

Grade 2 : Power detectable only with gravity.

Grade 3 : Limb can be held, against gravity but not against examiner's resistance.

Grade 4 : There is some degree of weakness. Usually described as poor or moderate strengths.

Grade 5 : Normal power is present.

Assessment is done by asking the patient to do a particular act and then tested by comparison with what he judges to be normal.

e.g. Rotators of the thigh: With the lower limb extended on the bed, ask the patient to roll it outwards and inwards against resistance.

IV. Reflexes

Integrated, involuntary neuro-muscular or motor responses to an adequate stimulus.

CLASSIFICATIONS

Somatic

1. **Superficial Reflexes (have their centres in higher regions of brain)**
   a. **The Plantar Reflex:** Assessment of the plantar reflex is of great clinical importance, not least because it is an objective response, which can be easily compared by various observers. To elicit it, the muscles of the lower limb should be relaxed. The outer edge of the sole of the foot is stimulated by gentle scratching a key or a pin along it from the heel towards the little toe and then medially across the metatarsus. In healthy adults even a slight stimulus produces a contraction of the tensor fascia lata often accompanied by a slighter contraction of the adductors of the thigh and of the sartorius. With a slightly stronger stimulus, flexion of the four toes appears, which increases with the strength of the stimulus till all the toes are flexed on the metatarsus and drawn together, the ankle being flexed and inverted. This is called the flexor plantar response. With still stronger stimuli withdrawal of the limb occurs. It is doubtful that the plantar reflex is ever completely absent in healthy subjects. The character of this reflex changes (becomes dorsiflexion) in upper motor

neuronal lesion. This sign of upgoing toe and dorsiflexion of ankle is known as Babinski's sign.

b. **Superficial Abdominal Reflexes:** These are elicited by allowing the patient to lie, relaxed and in a supine position, with the abdomen uncovered. A light stimulus, such as a key or a thin wooden stick, is passed across the abdominal skin in the plane of the dermatome from the outer aspect towards the midline. A ripple of contraction of the underlying abdominal musculature follows the stimulus. These reflexes are absent in upper motor neuron lesions above their spinal level. In disease of the thoracic spine they may indicate the segmental level of the lesion by their absence below this level.
   It is often impossible to obtain them in anxious patients, in the elderly or obese and in multiparous women.

2. **Deep Reflexes: (Also known as stretch or mono-synaptic reflexes)**

   a. **Knee Jerk:** The knee jerk is the best known of the tendon reflexes. The patellar hammer derives its name from its invention as an instrument for eliciting this reflex, the first tendon reflex consists of a contraction of the quadriceps when the patellar tendon is tapped. The spinal segments concerned are the 2nd, 3rd and 4th lumbar. It is best tested with the patient supine. The examiner's hand is passed under the knee to be tested or leg is placed upon the opposite knee, the knee to be tested rests on the dorsum of the observer's wrist. The patellar tendon is struck midway between its origin and insertion. Following the blow there will be brief extension of the knee from contraction of the quadriceps. The reflex can sometimes be more easily elicited with the patient sitting up, his legs dangling freely over the edge of the bed.
   The briskness of the knee jerk varies greatly in different individuals. In health it is hardly ever entirely absent. Sometimes, as in the case of the other tendon reflexes, one is unable to elicit it without applying reinforcement (Jendrassik's maneuver). This is done by asking the patient to make some strong voluntary muscular effort with the upper limbs, for example to hook the fingers of the two hands together and then to pull them against one another as hard as possible. While he is doing this, a further attempt is made to elicit the knee jerk.
   Reinforcement acts by increasing the sensitivity of the muscle spindle primary sense endings to stretch (by increased gamma fusimotor drive).

   b. **Ankle Jerk:** Place the lower limb on the bed so that it lies everted and slightly flexed. Then, with one hand, slightly dorsiflex the foot as to stretch the Achilles tendon and, with the other hand, strike the tendon on its posterior surface. A sharp contraction of the calf muscles results. This reflex can also be conveniently elicited when the patient is kneeling on a chair. It depends upon the 1st and 2nd sacral segments.

   c. **Triceps Jerk:** Flex the elbow and allow the forearm to rest across the patient's chest. Tap the triceps tendon just above the olecranon. The triceps contracts. The reflex depends upon the 6th and 7th cervical segments. Care must be taken to strike the triceps tendon and not the belly of the muscle itself. All muscles show a certain amount of irritability to direct mechanical stimuli; but this is a direct response, not a stretch reflex.

   d. **Biceps Jerk:** The elbow is flexed to a right angle and the forearm placed in a semipronated position the examiner then places his thumb on index finger on the biceps tendon and strikes it with the patellar hammer. The biceps contracts. The 5th and 6th cervical segments of the cord are concerned.

   e. **Supinator Jerk:** A blow upon the styloid process of the radius streteches the supinator causing supination of the elbow. This reflex depends on the 5th and 6th cervical segments.
   With lesions at this level the supinator reflex may be lost but, when it is tested, brisk flexion of the fingers is seen. This phenomenon is known as inversion of the reflex and it is evidence of hyper-excitability of the anterior horn cells below $C_{5/6}$ level. The reponsible lesion is in the $C_{5/6}$.

   f. **Jaw Jerk:** Ask the patient to open his mouth, but not too widely. Place one finger firmly on his chin and then tap it suddenly with the other hand as in percussion. A contraction of the muscles that close the jaw results. The jerk is sometimes absent in health and is increased in upper motor neuron lesions above the 5th nerve nuclei.

Autonomic (Response involves ANS arch)

E.g. Gag reflex or swallowing reflex.

Grading the Reflexes

Grade 0 : Absent (as in lower motor neuron type of lesions).
Grade 2: Brisk (as a normal knee jerk).
Grade 3: Very brisk (as in upper motor neuron type of lesions).
Grade 4: Clonus (as in upper motor neuron type of lesions).

V Coordination

By this is meant the smooth recruitment, interaction and cooperation of separate muscles or groups of muscles, in order to accomplish a definite motor act.

Finger Nose Test

Ask the patient to touch the point of his nose, first with one forefinger and then with the other.

VI. Gait

With the legs exposed and feet bare the patient is asked to walk away from the observer, to turn around at a given point and then to come towards him again. Observe the patient's walk.

Note: (1) If he can walk.

(2) If he can walk in a straight line or if he deviates to one side or another.

If he has a tendency to fall and if so in what direction.

VII. Involuntary Movements

These are unintended movements at rest or during voluntary movement. This can be detected by observing the patient during rest or while performing some act. E.g. tremors and tics.

Superficial Reflexes

	Right side	*Left side*
Plantar Reflex		
Abdominal Reflex		
Corneal Reflex		
Conjunctival Reflex		
Pupillary Reflex		
Cremasteric		

Deep Reflexes

Upper Extremity

	Right side	*Left side*
Biceps Jerk		
Triceps Jerk		
Supinator Jerk (brachioradialis)		

Lower Extremity

	Right side	*Left side*
Ankle jerks		
Knee jerks		

Table 31.1: Motor function

Nutrition

	Right	*Left*
Upper Extremity		
5" above elbow		
4" below elbow		
Lower Extremity		
9" above knee		
6" below elbow		

Table 31.2

Tone	*Normal*		*Increased tone (Hypertonia)*		*Decreased tone (Hypotonia)*	
	Right side	*Left side*	*Right side*	*Left side*	*Right side*	*Left side*
Upper Extremity						
i. Degree of Resistance						
ii. Type of Resistance						
iii. Range of Movement						
Lower Extremity						
i. Degree of Resistance						
ii. Type of Resistance						
iii. Range of Movement						

Table 31.3: Muscle power

Muscle Powers *Muscle Groups*	*Grade of Muscle Power*
Neck flexors and extensors	
Shoulder girdle (movement of the arm forwards, to the side and over the head)	
Upper arm muscles (Flexion and extension of elbow mainly)	
Forearm muscle (Flexion extension of the wrist, pronation, supination of the forearm)	
Finger movements (Flexion, extension, adduction and abduction)	
Abdominal muscle (Tested by raising head on legs in supine position)	
Hip girdle (Flexion, extension, abduction)	
Thigh muscles (Extension and flexion of knee)	
Leg muscles (Dorsiflexion, plantar flexion, eversion and inversion of foot)	

Table 31.4

Co-ordination	*Co-ordination*	
	Right	Left
Upper Extremity		
Finger Nose Test		
Finger to Finger Test		
Lower Extremity		
Knee Heel Test		
Romberg's Test		

Table 31.5: Abnormal movements

Generalised	
Localised	
Type	

Questions:

1. What are the different clinical conditions giving rise to atrophy and hypertrophy of skeletal muscles?
2. What is clasp knife spasticity? In which clinical disorder it is observed?
3. What is lead pipe and cogwheel rigidity? In which clinical condition it is observed?
4. Enumerate the clinical conditions which give rise to hypotonia of the muscles.
5. What are the tests for rigidity in meningitis?
6. Give root values of the reflexes you have tested in a tabular form.
7. What is the state of superficial and deep reflexes in UMN and LMN lesions.
8. Name the brain regions concerned with (i) co-ordination of movements (ii) gait and speech.
9. Give examples of mono and polysynaptic reflexes.

EXAMINATION OF SENSORY SYSTEM

AIM

To test sensory functions of human subjects. (Assess functional integrity of specific sensory pathways, i.e., spino-thalamic and luminiscal system).

REQUISITES

Cotton wool, pins, test tubes containing hot and cold water, Weber's compass, different sizes of matchsticks and tuning fork.

PROCEDURE

In investigating the sensory functions of a subject, we have to test the acuteness of the following **forms of sensitivity**.

1. **Tactile sensibility:** This includes the powers of appreciating light touch and pressure, and of tactile localisation and discrimination.
2. The sense of position and the appreciation of passive movements.
3. The recognition of the size, shape, weight and form of objects.
4. The appreciation of vibration.
5. Sensibility to pain.
6. Thermal sensibility.
7. In addition the presence or absence of any abnormal sensation is also noted.

At the outset explain to the patient the tests to be performed and so secure as far as possible his intelligent cooperation. The eyes should then be closed, and the different forms of sensibility tested as follows:

1. **Tactile Sensibilty**

   Use a wisp of cotton wool or fine camel hairbrush. If it is desired to test the sensibility of the skin to light touch, over a hairy part, it is essential to shave it, as the sensibility of the hairs themselves is so acute.

   Appreciation of light touch and pressure, and of tactile localisation

   Tell the subject to say **"Now"** every time he feels a touch. Compare corresponding points on opposite sides of the body and employ every now and then a negative test, asking the subject if he feels your touch, in order to prevent him making random replies. The appreciation of pressure touch should then be tested. This may be done by touching him with the tip of your finger or any blunt object. It is important that its temperature should not differ much from that of the skin, and the pressure must not be so heavy as to give pain or discomfort. Ask him also to localise the stimulus by describing or in any way indicating the exact position of the spot touched. This is important, as a subject may be able to feel the stimulus and not be able to localise it.

   Tactile Discrimination: The ability to discriminate between two points is tested with Weber's compasses. The subject is asked whether he is being touched with one or both points of the compass. The points of the Weber's compass are first separated wide enough for the subject to be able to appreciate them as two points and then gradually brought closer together. Normally 1 cm of separation of the points is appreciated on the palmar surfaces of the thumb and fingers.

2. **Sense of Position and Appreciation of Passive Movements**

   The subject's eyes being carefully shut, take hold of one of his limbs and move it about in various directions through the air, finally leaving it in some definite positions, say semi-flexed and slightly elevated, then ask him to put the other corresponding limb in a similar position.

The appreciation of movement is closely related to the sense of position, and should be tested at the same time. Grasp any segment of a limb firmly, and then move it gradually into another position, ask the subject to say "NOW" as soon as he recognises the movement and note the angle through which the limb was moved, for him to be able to recognize movement.

Finally test that the patient can recognize the direction of the movement, that is, whether the joint is flexed or extended.

3. **The Recognition of Size, Shape and Form**

These faculties can be tested most accurately in the hands. To test size, place in the subject's palm, objects of the same shape, but of different sizes such as small rods or matchsticks of different length. The two objects should be applied consecutively, and he is asked to say which is the larger.

To test the power of recognising form, familiar objects, such as coins, a pencil, a penknife, scissors etc. are placed in the hand, and the subject is asked to identify them or to describe their form.

4. **Appreciation of Vibration**

If the foot of a vibrating tuning fork is placed on the surface of the body the vibrations can be felt provided they are sufficiently strong. This is a valuable test, as the ability to appreciate vibration may be lost in various diseases, such as tabes dorsalis, peripheral neuritis, and conditions that involve the posterior columns of the cord. A heavy tuning fork of 128 vibrations per second is generally employed. Make the fork vibrate by striking its prongs gently on a firm object, and place its foot immediately on the part to be tested. Ascertain if the subject perceives the vibrations, and if so. Ask him to say at once when he ceases to feel them. If the fork is then transferred to the observer, it can be seen if the sensibility to the vibration is diminished or not, and the amount of diminution can be measured by the further time that the vibration can be perceived by the normal person.

5. **Sensibility to Pain**

Pain may be evoked either by a cutaneous stimulus, as the prick of a pin or by pressure on the deeper structures, such as the muscles or bones. Sensibility to superficial and to pressure pain should be tested separately.

A. Superficial Pain: The point of a steel pin should be used as a stimulus. Care must be taken that the patient distinguishes between the sharpness of the point (that is, its relative size) and the pain which the prick evokes, it often happens that even when sensibility to pain is abolished he can recognise that the stimulus is pointed, and thus confuse the observer by calling it "sharp".

B. Pressure Pain is examined by squeezing the muscles or the tendoachilles.

6. **Thermal Sensibility**

This is conveniently examined by using test tubes containing hot and cold water. The part to be tested is touched with each in turn, and the subject says whether each tube is hot or cold. It is often important to determine the thresholds for hot and cold i.e. the lowest temperature that is warm and the highest that is cold. This can be done by noting the temperature of the water in the tubes.

7. Look for any **abnormal sensation** if present.

Examination of Sensory System

Name

Age

Sex

Symptoms

1. Pain
2. Tingling and numbness
3. Anesthesia
4. Analgesia
5. Thermoanesthesia

Physical Examination–Testing the Sensations

Superficial

1. Tactile sensibility
2. Tactile localisation
3. Tactile discrimination
4. Temperature
5. Pain

Deep

1. Deep sensation
2. Deep pressure
3. Position of joint
4. Vibration
5. Deep pain
6. Appreciation of movement

32

COLD PRESSOR TEST

PRINCIPLE

Under condition of stress of either physical or psychological origin, there is activation of sympathetic nervous system. The cold pressor response consists of placing the hand into cold water as painful stimulus. This is used to study the autonomic response. The afferent fibers for this response are pain fibers and the efferent fibers are sympathetic fibers.

Normally there is a rise of more than 10 mm of Hg in systolic B.P.

PROCEDURE

1. Explain the procedure to the subject to allay anxiety or apprehension.
2. Record the resting blood pressure with the subject sitting comfortably.
3. The subject is asked to immerse the hand in the cold water at a temperature of 4-6°C for 2 minutes.
4. B.P. is recorded at every 30 seconds.
5. After 2 minutes the subject is asked to remove his hand out of the water.
6. Measure the B.P.
7. Calculate the increase in systolic B.P.

Observations and Results

	Systolic B.P.	*Diastolic B.P.*
Basal or resting		
During		
I		
II		
III		
IV		
After		

Calculate

Increase in BP = Maximal systolic BP during – Basal BP

Questions:

1. How is the systolic and diastolic blood pressure varying with cold stress?
2. How would you explain these changes physiologically?
3. What is the clinical significance of this test?
4. In which conditions are the cold pressor response blunted or abnormal?

33 RECORDING TEMPERATURE

RECORDING OF BODY TEMPERATURE AND THE EFFECT OF EXERCISE

AIM

To record the body temperature with the help of a clinical thermometer and to observe the effect of exercise on it.

PRINCIPLE

Mercury expands on being heated and the expansion is proportional to the rise in temperature.

REQUISITES

Clinical thermometer, container of any antiseptic solution, running water.

Clinical Thermometer

It contains a glass bulb, which has mercury inside it and a capillary limb. The capillary limb has graduations marked from 95°F to 108°/110° F. At the junction of the main bulb with the capillary limb there is a constriction (twist), which does not let the mercury slide down once it has risen. A good thermometer has a curved surface, which acts as a lens and magnifies the width of the mercury. It also has a flattened back, which is painted white against which the index can be read with ease.

PROCEDURE

- Clean the thermometer by dipping for 30 sec. in antiseptic solution and then wash under running water.
- Bring down the mercury by shaking the thermometer.
- The thermometer should be placed in a site where the tissues of the body completely surround the bulb. The positions available are the mouth, armpit, vagina and rectum. The fold of the groin with the thigh flexed is used in infants. Whatever skin site is selected the part coming in contact with the thermometer must be dry, clean and unexposed to the surroundings.
- When the temperature is taken in the mouth, the bulb is placed under the tongue with the lips closed about the stem and the patient is asked to breathe through the nose. Hot or cold drinks taken prior to the reading are likely to affect the temperature.
- If axilla is selected, it should be cleaned with a towel and the bulb must be placed deeply in the hollow of the armpit and the arm brought well across the chest. No fold of clothing should come in between the skin and the thermometer.

Time

All thermometers are marked '½ minute' as the period for which they are required to be kept in position, but they should be kept for at least a minute.

PRECAUTIONS

- Take three readings and take the average of the three.
- Take the reading immediately after removing the thermometer, through the curved surface and against the flat white background.
- After the use the thermometer should be cleaned with water and sterilized with the rectified spirit or any antiseptic solution.
- Take the temperature both in the mouth and in the axilla. The mouth temperature is ½ to 1 degree higher than the axillary temperature.

To See the Effect of Exercise on Body Temperature

After taking the basal readings, do a 5-minute vigorous exercise and take the temperature immediately on completion of exercise and after every 2 minutes till readings return to normal.

Basal

Oral temperature	*Axillary temperature*
1	
2	
3	

Mean Body Temperature

After 5 Minutes Exercise

	Oral temperature
Immediately after exercise	
After 2 min.	
After 4 min.	
After 6 min.	

Questions:

1. What is the normal body temperature? What is hyperpyrexia?
2. List the various causes of physiological variation in body temperature.
3. List the pathological causes of a rise in body temperature.
4. What are the physiological mechanisms activated by exposure to heat and cold?
5. What is core temperature of the body?
6. Recording of temperature from which sites of the body is likely to reflect core temperature?
7. Name the brain structures concerned with body temperature regulation.

34 ELECTROMYOGRAPHY AND NERVE CONDUCTION VELOCITY (EMG and NCV)

HISTORICAL BASIS

The first documented experiments dealing with EMG started with Francesco Redi's works in 1666. Redi discovered a highly specialized muscle of the electric ray fish (Electric Eel) generated electricity. By 1773, Walsh had been able to demonstrate that the Eel fish's muscle tissue could generate a spark of electricity. In 1792, a publication entitled *De Viribus Electricitatis in Motu Musculari Commentarius* appeared, written by Luigi Galvani, in which the author demonstrated that electricity could initiate muscle contractions. Six decades later, in 1849, Emil du Bois-Reymond discovered that it was also possible to record electrical activity during a voluntary muscle contraction. The first actual recording of this activity was made by Marey in 1890, who also introduced the term electromyography. In 1922, Gasser and Erlanger used an oscilloscope to show the electrical signals from muscles. Because of the stochastic nature of the myoelectric signal, only rough information could be obtained from its observation. The capability of detecting electromyographic signals improved steadily from the 1930s through the 1950s, and researchers began to use improved electrodes more widely for the study of muscles. Clinical use of surface EMG (sEMG) for the treatment of more specific disorders began in the 1960s. Hardyck and his researchers were the first (1966) practitioners to use sEMG. In the early 1980s, Cram and Steger introduced a clinical method for scanning a variety of muscles using an EMG sensing device.

It is not until the middle of the 1980s that integration techniques in electrodes had sufficiently advanced to allow batch production of the required small and lightweight instrumentation and amplifiers. At present, a number of suitable amplifiers are commercially available. In the early 1980s, cables that produced signals in the desired microvolt range became available. Recent research has resulted in a better understanding of the properties of surface EMG recording. Surface electromyography is increasingly used for recording from superficial muscles in clinical or kinesiological protocols, where intramuscular electrodes are used for investigating deep muscles or localized muscle activity.

INTRODUCTION

Electromyography refers to recording of action potentials of muscle fibers firing singly or in groups near the needle electrode in a muscle. The muscle action potential when recorded by a needle appears triphasic as the action potential approaches, crosses, and leaves the recording electrode. Recording from an area incapable of propagating the impulse, therefore, results in a large positivity with a low and long negativity. The distance of recording electrode from the muscle fibers determines the rise time and fall of muscle action potential. The normal muscle fibers are under neural control. The rate and pattern of firing of the muscle fibers of a motor unit, therefore, depends on the stimuli approaching through the nerve. The denervated muscle fibers on the other hand have unstable membrane potential and fire spontaneously (without stimulation), individually (single fiber) and regularly

Equipment

The basic equipment for EMG consist of electrodes a high gain amplifier with a selectivity for frequencies from about 10 to 500 Hz, and an arrangement for recording the output

Types of EMG Needle Electrodes (Fig. 34.1)

A. Needle Electrode

1. Concentric needle electrode.
2. Monopolar needle electrode.
3. Single fiber (SF) needle electrode.
4. Macro electrode.

B. Surface Electrode

The amplifier is commonly a part of an EMG machine which also includes an ink recorder. The ink recorder is convenient but not ideal for the higher frequency EMG signals. For a

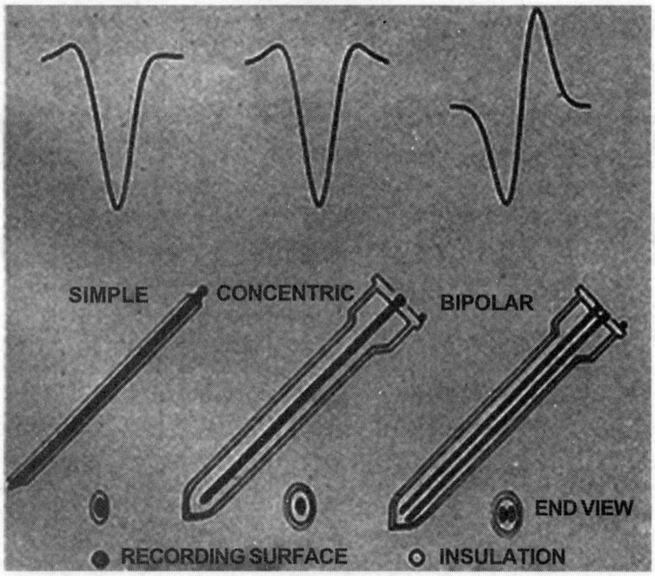

Fig. 34.1: Three types of EMG needles and records that could be used to record the same extracellular voltage changes associated with an action potential

more faithful recording of the higher frequencies, the amplifier may be connected to an oscilloscope. The oscilloscopic traces may be photographed or stored on magnetic tape. In addition, the EMG signals may be fed to an audio unit for an on the spot feel of the signals. Finally the EMG is best done in a specially constructed shielded room to prevent interference due to extraneous electromagnetic and electrostatic forces.

Recording Technique

The equipment setup for EMG recordings is as follows: sweep speed 5-10 ms/div; amplification 50 μV/division for MUPs and filter setting 20-10000 Hz. The duration of MUPs should be measured at a gain of 100 μV/div and sweep speed of 5 ms/div and low filter at 2-3 Hz. Almost every muscle in body can be studied with needle EMG. This, however, is neither desirable nor practical; therefore, for each study, a balance must be achieved between studying a sufficient number of muscles to reach or exclude a diagnosis. Patient's cooperation is important for proper interpretation of EMG, therefore, they should be properly explained about the test. For EMG of each muscle the following steps should be followed:

1. Select the muscle.
2. Instruct the patient how to contract and relax the muscle.
3. Identify the muscle while patient is contracting and relaxing the muscle.
4. Locate the needle insertion point slightly away from the motor point to prevent endplate noise.

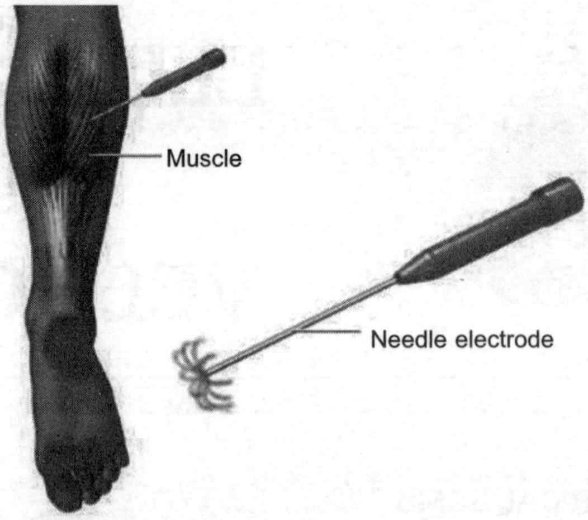

Fig. 34.2

5. Insert the needle quickly while the muscle is relaxed to minimize the pain.
6. Sharp MUPs on minimal contraction conform that the needle is in proper position. If MUPs are not sharp, needle should be repositioned.

In needle EMG, following three types of activities are studied:

1. Insertional activity.
2. Spontaneous activity.
3. Voluntary activities.

Insertional Activity

Introduction of the needle into the muscle normally produces a brief burst of electrical activity due to mechanical damage by needle movement and it lasts slightly exceeding the needle movement (0.5–1s). Increased insertional activity is defined as any activity other than endplate potential lasting more than 300 ms after brief needle movement.

Spontaneous Activity

Once the insertional activity decays after a second or so, in normal individuals, there is no spontaneous electrical activity.

The abnormal spontaneous activities include the following:

A. Spontaneous activities originated from muscle fiber

1. Fibrillations and positive sharp waves.
2. Myotonic discharges.
3. Complex repetitive discharges (CRD).

B. Spontaneous activities originated from motor neuron or axon

1. Fasciculations.
2. Doublets, triplets and multiplets.
3. Myokymia.
4. Neuromyotonia.
5. Cramps.

ABNORMAL SPONTANEOUS ACTIVITIES ORIGINATING FROM MUSCLE FIBER

Fibrillations and Positive Sharp Waves

Fibrillations are spontaneously occurring action potentials from a single muscle fiber. Fibrillation fires regularly at a rate of 0.5-15 Hz, with an amplitude of 20-200 μV and duration of 1-5 ms when recorded by a concentric needle. Fibrillations may rarely be irregular; however, in such a situation the inter-spike interval exceeds 70 ms. Fibrillations are biphasic or triphasic waves with initial positivity, which is an important differentiating feature from endplate spike.

Myotonic Discharges

The action potentials of muscle fibers firing for a prolonged period after external excitation are the characteristic of myotonic discharges. The action potentials wax and wan in amplitude and frequency because of muscle membrane abnormality. The myotonic discharges are rhythmic with frequency ranging between 20 Hz and 150 Hz. The variation in frequency gives rise to a sound like a dive–bomber.

ABNORMAL SPONTANEOUS ACTIVITIES ORIGINATING FROM MOTOR NEURON OR AXONS

Fasciculations

Fasciculations potential are spontaneous contractions of a number of muscle fibers belonging to a whole or a part of motor unit. Fasciculations occur randomly and irregularly at variable rates ranging between 0.1 Hz and 10 Hz. The size and shape of fasciculations depend on the motor unit from which they arise and to the distance of recording electrode from the motor unit. Fasciculations may have the appearance of normal or abnormal MUP and can be recognized by their slower firing rate compared to MUP.

NORMAL MOTOR UNIT POTENTIAL

After evaluation of insertional and spontaneous activity, the next step of needle EMG is evaluation of MUP on voluntary contraction. The basic unit of peripheral nervous system is the motor unit, which comprises individual lower motor neuron, its axon, neuromuscular junction (NMJ), and muscle fibers. The number of muscle fibers in a motor unit varies from 9 in extra ocular muscles to 1900 in gastrocnemius.

The recruitment of motor unit following voluntary contraction is determined by size principle. The size of a motor unit is dependent on size of motor neuron, diameter of axon, thickness of myelin, conduction velocity, depolarization threshold, and metabolic type of muscle fiber. The larger motor neuron has larger axon and thicker myelin, hence faster conduction velocity, depolarization threshold, and metabolic type of muscle fiber and usually supplies Type II muscle fibers, which are required for fast twitch. On the other hand, small sized motor neurons has smaller axons and thinner myelin, hence slower conduction velocity, lower threshold for depolarization, and supplies Type I muscle fibers required for slow twitch.

According to size principle, the motor neurons are recruited from smallest to largest following voluntary contraction. In routine EMG most MUP analysed are the smaller low threshold representing Type I muscle fiber. This explains that EMG in most metabolic myopathies including steroid myopathy is normal as these primarily affect the Type II fibers.

MUP represents the sum of the action potentials supplied by an anterior horn cell.

CLINICAL IMPORTANCE

EMG signals are used in many clinical and biomedical applications. EMG is used as a diagnostics tool for identifying neuromuscular diseases, assessing low-back pain, kinesiology, and disorders of motor control. EMG signals are also used as a control signal for prosthetic devices such as prosthetic hands, arms, and lower limbs. In neuropathies the MUP duration (5 ms to 15 ms) and amplitude are normal (0.1 mv to 2 mv) however the recruitment firing pattern is reduced e.g. acute demyelinating diseases, amyotropic lateral sclerosis. In myopathies the MUP duration and amplitude is reduced and the recruitment firing pattern is also reduced e.g. spinal muscular atrophy.

Normal Pattern of EMG

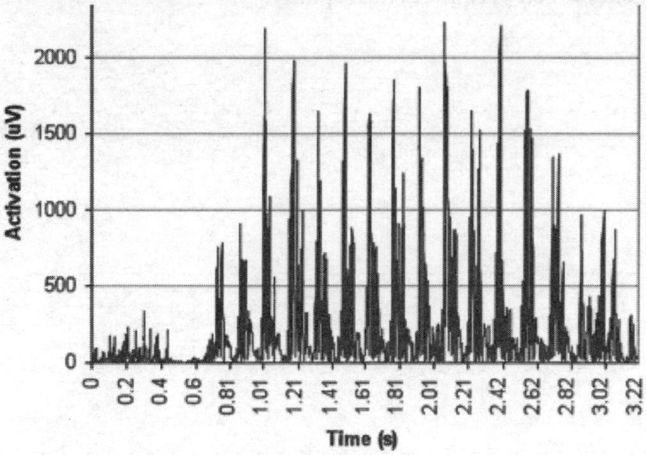

Fig. 34.3

Recruitment of Motor Units

Motor unit potential is normal in acute denervation, becomes polyphasic and of long duration during reinervation because of collateral sprouting and fiber grouping. The MUP becomes polyphasic and of short duration because of muscle necrosis and fiber splitting in myopathies.

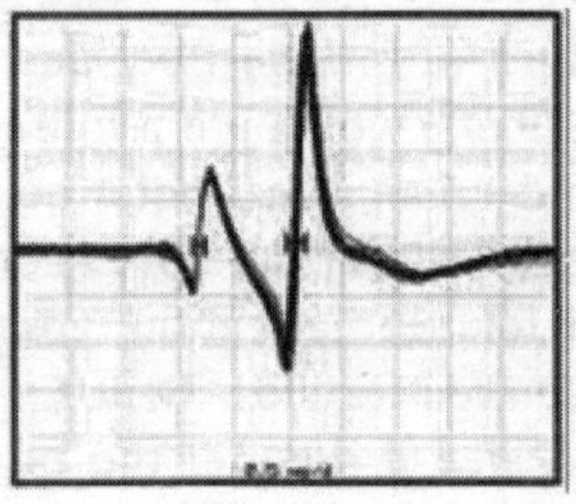

Fig. 34.4

NERVE CONDUCTION VELOCITY (NCV)

Nerve conduction velocity (NCV) test is a measurement of the speed of conduction of an electrical impulse through a nerve. NCV can determine nerve damage and destruction.

During the test, the nerve is stimulated, usually with surface electrode patches attached to the skin. Two electrodes are placed on the skin over the nerve. One electrode stimulates the nerve with a very mild electrical impulse and the other electrode records it. The resulting electrical activity is recorded by another electrode. This is repeated for each nerve being tested.

The nerve conduction velocity (speed) is then calculated by measuring the distance between electrodes and the time it takes for electrical impulses to travel between electrodes.

Slowing of the NCV usually indicates there is damage to the myelin. Another example, slowing across the wrist for the motor and sensory latencies of the median nerve indicates focal compression of the median nerve at the wrist, called carpal tunnel syndrome. On the other hand, slowing of all nerve conductions in more than one limb indicates generalized diseased nerves, or generalized peripheral neuropathy. People with diabetes mellitus often develop generalized peripheral neuropathy.

F-wave study

F-wave study uses supramaximal stimulation of a motor nerve and recording of action potentials from a muscle supplied by the nerve. This is not a reflex, per se, in that the action potential travels from the site of the stimulating electrode in the limb to the spinal cord's ventral horn and back to the limb in the same nerve that was stimulated. The F-wave latency can be used to derive the conduction velocity of nerve between the limb and spine, whereas the motor and sensory nerve conduction studies evaluate conduction in the segment of the limb.

H-reflex study

H-reflex study uses stimulation of a nerve and recording the reflex electrical discharge from a muscle in the limb. This also evaluates conduction between the limb and the spinal cord, but in this case, the afferent impulses (those going toward the spinal cord) are in sensory nerves while the efferent impulses (those coming from the spinal cord) are in motor nerves.

Questions:

1. What is motor unit? What is the normal amplitude and duration of a motor unit potential?
2. What are the types of electrodes used in EMG?
3. What is insertional activity?
4. Enumerate the uses of EMG.
5. How is nerve conduction velocity calculated?
6. What is H reflex?

35

ELECTROENCEPHALOGRAPHY

Electroencephalogram is the record of repetitive electrical waves due to summation of postsynaptic potentials of many hundred thousands neurons.

SOURCE OF EEG ACTIVITY

EEG is the summated synaptic activity of a very large number of pyramidal cells in the cortex. EEG activity originates in thalamocortical dipoles. EEG activity therefore always reflects the summation of the *synchronous activity* of thousands or millions of neurons that have similar spatial orientation. If the cells do not have similar spatial orientation, their ions do not line up and create waves to be detected. The electrical activity is measured at the surface. This process is known as volume conduction.

EEG RECORDING TECHNIQUE

In conventional scalp EEG, the recording is obtained by placing electrodes on the scalp with a conductive gel or paste, usually after preparing the scalp area by light abrasion to reduce impedance due to dead skin cells. Many systems typically use electrodes, each of which is attached to an individual wire.

Each electrode is connected to one input of a differential amplifier (one amplifier per pair of electrodes). These amplifiers amplify the voltage between the active electrode and the reference (typically 1,000–100,000 times, or 60–100 dB of voltage gain).

During the recording, a series of activation procedures may be used. These procedures may induce normal or abnormal EEG activity that might not otherwise be seen. These procedures include hyperventilation, photic stimulation (with a strobe light), eye closure, mental activity, sleep and sleep deprivation. During (inpatient) epilepsy monitoring, a patient's typical seizure medications may be withdrawn.

A typical adult human EEG signal is about 10μV to 100 μV in amplitude when measured from the scalp.

ELECTRODE PLACEMENT

The **10-20 system** or **International 10-20 system** is an internationally recognized method to describe and apply the location of scalp electrodes in the context of an EEG test or experiment. This method was developed by the International Federation of Societies for Electroencephalography and Clinical Neurophysiology. The system is based upon measurement from four standard points on the head: the nasion, the inion, and the left and right preauricular points. The "10" and "20" refer to the fact that the electrodes are spaced either 10% or 20% of the total distance between a given pair of skull landmarks i.e nasion to inion. This helps to standardise the recording throughout the world as it is consistent for every patient.

Each site has a letter to identify the lobe and a number to identify the hemisphere location. The letters F, T, C, P and O stand for frontal, temporal, central, parietal, and occipital lobes, respectively. Note that there exists no central lobe, the "C" letter is only used for identification purposes only. A "z" (zero) refers to an electrode placed on the midline. Even numbers (2,4,6,8) refer to electrode positions on the right hemisphere, whereas odd numbers (1,3,5,7) refer to those on the left hemisphere.

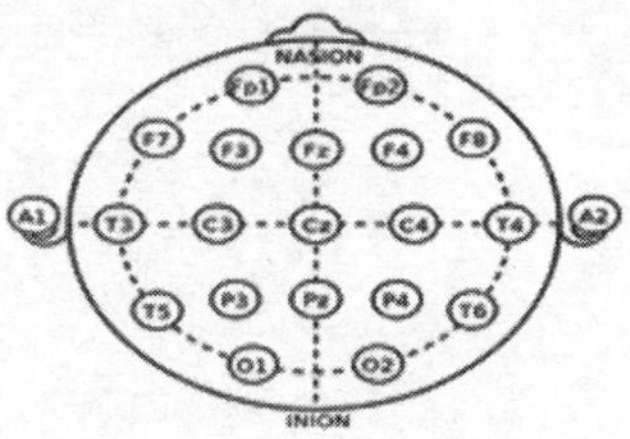

Fig. 35.1: 10-20 system or international 10-20 system

SPECTRAL ANALYSIS

Fourier power spectral analysis is done to smoothen the bar spectrum and predominant frequency in the EEG appears as a series of tall peaks. The frequency corresponding to the tallest peaks gives the EEG rhythm during recording.

EEG WAVES

In adult human beings who are awake but at rest, relaxed, with eyes closed and mind wandering, the predominant

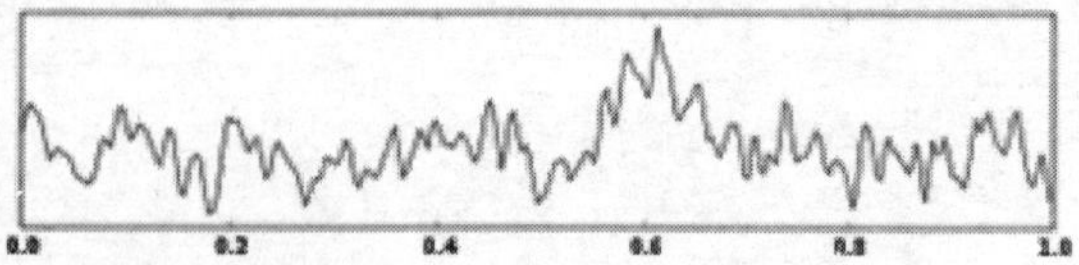

Fig. 35.2: Normal activity

EEG wave pattern is that of alpha rhythm (frequency of 8–13 Hz and amplitude 50–100 µv). This alpha rhythm is most marked in the parietal and occipital lobes and is related to decreased level of attention. When alpha is being generated, subjects report that they are relaxed and happy. However, people who normally experience more alpha than usual are not psychologically different from those with less alpha rhythm. Meditators and yoga practitioners may show more alpha actvity.

When attention is focused on something or a person is attentive to external stimulus or thinking hard or involved in arithmetic, the alpha rhythm is replaced by irregular low amplitude, high frequency beta rhythm (13–30 Hz). This phenomenon is called alpha block or arousal or alerting response or desynchronization as it represents breaking up of the obviously synchronized neural activity necessary to produce regular waves. Sometimes gamma oscillations at 30–80 Hz are seen on individual's arousal and focusing or attending to something in the ambient environment.

Hence it seems that frequency of EEG waves denote attention; more the attention, higher the frequency reflecting desynchronization. On decreasing the attention, EEG pattern reverts to alpha rhythm.

Delta waves, 100 µV, upto 4 Hz are seen in babies, during slow wave sleep in adults.

Theta waves, 10 µV, 4-8 Hz is seen in young children, during idling, drowsiness in older children and adults.

CLINICAL USE

A routine clinical EEG recording typically lasts 20–30 minutes (plus preparation time). Variations in EEG waves (frequency, morphology and seizure potentials) can be of diagnostic value in certain diseases.

Routine EEG is typically used in the following clinical circumstances:

- To distinguish *epileptic seizures* from other types of spells, such as *psychogenic non-epileptic seizures*, *syncope (fainting)*, sub-cortical *movement disorders* and *migraine* variants. Epilepsy is associated with distincive high amplitude wave patterns known as spikes (upto 1000 µV) .
- To differentiate "organic" *encephalopathy* or *delirium* from primary psychiatric syndromes such as *catatonia*. General changes such as slowing and irregularity in the recorded curves accompany diffuse brain disease, cerebral trauma, coma.
- To serve as an adjunct test of *brain death*, as an isoelectric or flat EEG is being taken as a criteria for death. Other features of brain stem hypoxia include absence of light response, mydriasis (dialated fixed pupils), atonia and areflexia, unresposnsiveness.

Questions:

1. What is EEG?
2. What is the physiological basis of EEG genesis?
3. What is the importance of ARAS in synchronizing and desynchronizing the EEG?
4. Explain 10-20 system of electrode placement.
5. Give description of waves giving their frequency and amplitude.
6. What are the clinical implications of EEG?

36 EVOKED POTENTIALS

An **evoked potential** (or "evoked response") is a surface *electrical potential* recorded in response to a specific and adequate stimulus-auditory, visual or somatosensory. While EEG is the spontaneous electrical activity recorded from the surface of the scalp.

Evoked potential evoked by the stimulus (signal) have *amplitudes* that tend to be low, and is barely discernible amidst the backdrop of EEG waves. To resolve these low-amplitude potentials against the background of ongoing EEG, ECG, EMG, and other biological signals and ambient noise, signal *averaging* is usually required to enhance the signal-to-noise ratio.

EVOKED POTENTIALS CLASSIFIED

Based on the type of stimulus, evoked potentials may be visual, auditory or somatosensory. Based on the latency of the response, evoked potentials are classified into stimulus related and event related potentials.

STIMULUS RELATED POTENTIALS

There are three kinds of evoked potentials in widespread clinical use: auditory evoked potentials, usually recorded from the scalp but originating at *brainstem* level; visual evoked potentials, and *somatosensory evoked potentials,* which are elicited by electrical stimulation of peripheral nerve. *Visual* evoked potentials elicited by a flashing light or changing pattern on a monitor; *auditory* evoked potentials by a click or tone stimulus presented through earphones) or by tactile or *somatosensory* evoked potential (SSEP) elicited by tactile or electrical stimulation of a sensory or mixed nerve in the *periphery*.

The response to a stimulus for example auditory consists of a series of waves or stimulus related potentials. This response may be divided into three sequential time periods: the early, mid and the long latency responses.

VISUAL EVOKED POTENTIAL (Fig. 36.1)

VEP Stimuli

The checkerboard and grating patterns use light and dark squares and stripes, respectively. These squares and stripes are equal in size and are presented to one at a time via a television or computer screen.

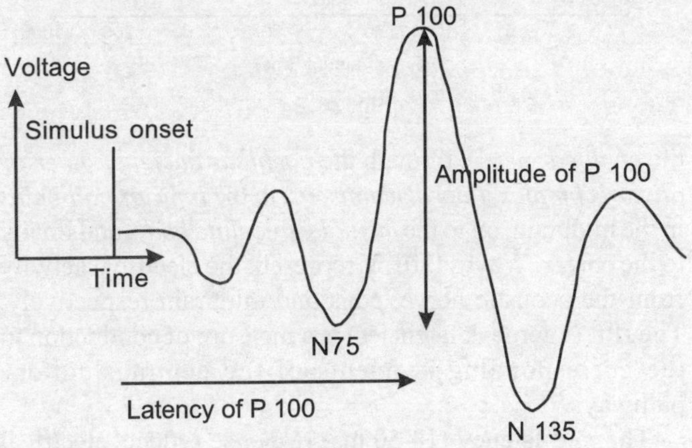

Fig. 36.1: The form of the VEP

VEP Electrode Placement

Electrode placement is extremely important to elicit a good VEP response free of artifact. One electrode is placed 2.5 cm above the inion and a reference electrode is placed at Fz. For a more detailed response, two additional electrodes can be placed 5 cm to the right and left of Oz.

VEP Waves

The VEP nomenclature is determined by using capital letters stating whether the peak is positive (P) or negative (N) followed by a number which indicates the average peak latency for that particular wave. For example, P50 is a wave with a positive peak at approximately 50 ms following stimulus onset.

The average amplitude for VEP waves usually falls between 5 and 10 microvolts.

AUDITORY EVOKED POTENTIAL (Fig. 36.2)

The early latecy (<10 ms) response is called Brainstem Auditory Evoked Potential (BAEP). The waves are named I to VI. These can be used to trace the signal generated by a sound through the ascending auditory pathway. The evoked potential is generated in the cochlea, goes through

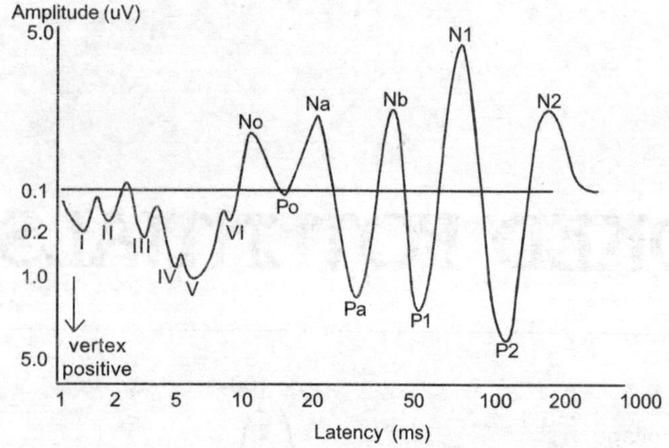

Fig. 36.2

the *cochlear nerve*, through the *cochlear nucleus*, *superior olivary complex*, *lateral lemniscus*, to the *inferior colliculus* in the midbrain, on to the *medial geniculate body*, and finally to the *cortex*. Waves I, III, V represent the electrical activity from the acoustic nerve, pons and midbrain respectively. The IPL (interpeak latencies) is a measure of conduction in the corresponding segments of the central auditory pathways.

The mid-latency (10-50 ms) response reflects electrical activity in the thalamocortical radiations, the primary auditory cortex and association cortex.

The neural generators of the long-latency (>50 ms) response are unknown. The response consists of a large negative wave (N1) and a large positive wave (P2). In the diagram above, these waves can be seen. They are also called slow vertex responses or vertex reponses as they can be elicited maximally at the vertex.

These waves represent the functional integrity of the CNS sensory pathway. They are largely independent of the subject's attention or level of arousal.

Somatosensory Evoked Potential

Somatosensory Evoked Potentials (SSEPs) are used in *neuromonitoring* to assess the function of a patient's *spinal cord* during *surgery*. They are recorded by stimulating peripheral nerves, most commonly the *tibial nerve*, *median nerve* or *ulnar nerve*, typically with an *electrical* stimulus. The response is then recorded from the patient's *scalp* (Fig. 36.3).

The two most looked at aspects of an SSEP are the amplitude and latency of the peaks. The most predominant peaks have been studied and named in labs. Each peak is given a letter and a number in its name. For example, N20 refers to a negative peak (N) at 20 ms. This peak is recorded from the cortex when the median nerve is stimulated. It most likely corresponds to the signal reaching the *somatosensory cortex*.

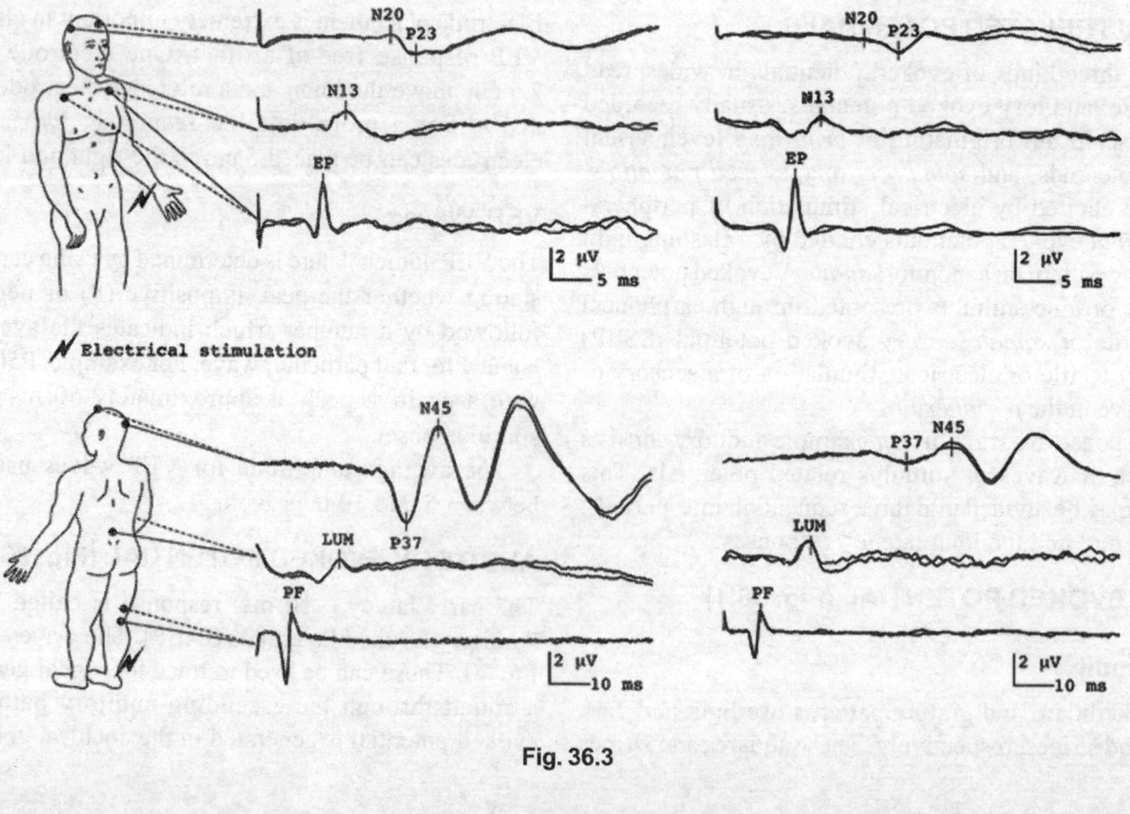

Fig. 36.3

Somatosensory evoked potentials provide monitoring for the dorsal columns of the spinal cord during surgeries which place brain structures at risk.

EVENT-RELATED POTENTIAL (Fig. 36.4)

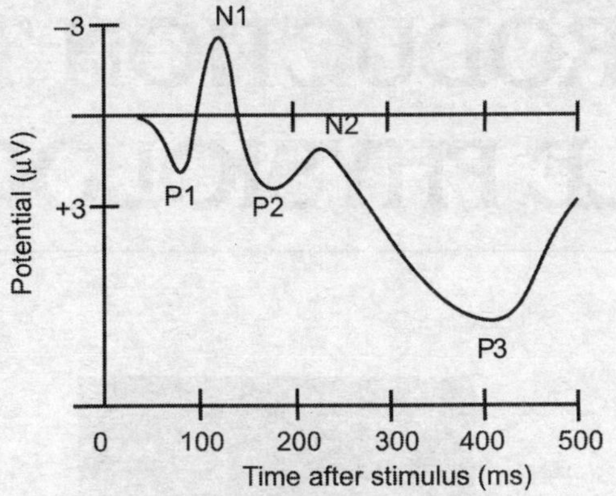

Fig. 36.4

A waveform showing several ERP components, including the *N100* and *P300*.

An event related potentials occur only when the patient is selectively attentive to the stimulus. The subject has to distinguish one stimulus (the target) from the other (the non targets).

The study of the brain in this way provides a *noninvasive* means of evaluating brain functioning in patients with cognitive diseases example assessment of dementia and delirium.

ERP COMPONENTS NOMENCLATURE

ERP waveforms consist of a series of positive and negative voltage deflections, called *components*. Though some ERP components are referred to with acronyms, most components are referred to by a letter (N/P) indicating polarity (negative/positive), followed by a number indicating either the latency in milliseconds. For instance, a negative-going peak that is the first substantial peak in the waveform and often occurs about 100 milliseconds after a stimulus is presented is often called the *N100* (indicating its latency is 100 ms after the stimulus and that it is negative) or N1 (indicating that it is the first peak and is negative); it is often followed by a positive peak, usually called the *P200* or P2. The stated latencies for ERP components are often quite variable. For example, the *P300* component may exhibit a peak anywhere between 250 ms - 700 ms.

While *evoked potentials* reflect the processing of the physical stimulus, event-related potentials are caused by the "higher" processes, that might involve *memory, expectation, attention,* or changes in the mental state, among others.

CLINICAL ERP

Physicians and *neurologists* will sometimes use a flashing *visual* checkerboard stimulus to test for any damage or trauma in the visual system. In a healthy person, this stimulus will elicit a strong response over the primary *visual cortex* located in the *occipital lobe,* in the back of the brain.

ERP component abnormalities in clinical research have been shown in neurological conditions such as:

- Dementia.
- Parkinson's disease.
- Multiple sclerosis.
- Head injuries.
- Stroke.

RESEARCH ERP

ERPs are used extensively in *neuroscience, cognitive psychology, cognitive science* and *psycho-physiological* research. *Experimental psychologists* and *neuroscientists* have discovered many different stimuli that elicit reliable ERPs from participants. The timing of these responses is thought to provide a measure of the timing of the brain's communication or timing of information processing. For example, in the checkerboard paradigm described above, healthy participants' first response of the visual cortex is around 50-70 ms. This would seem to indicate that this is the amount of time it takes for the *transduced* visual stimulus to reach the *cortex* after *light* first enters the *eye*. Alternatively, the *P300* response occurs at around 300 ms in the *oddball paradigm,* for example, regardless of the type of stimulus presented: *visual, tactile, auditory, olfactory, gustatory,* etc. Because of this general invariance with regard to stimulus type, the P300 component is understood to reflect a higher cognitive response to unexpected and/or cognitively *salient* stimuli.

Questions:

1. What are evoked potentials? Classify them.
2. Explain the significance of the waves of brainstem auditory evoked potential.
3. What are event related evoked potential?
4. Enumerate the uses of evoked potentials.

37

AMPHIBIAN EXPERIMENTS: INTRODUCTION TO NERVE-MUSCLE PHYSIOLOGY

For experiments in nerve-muscle physiology, frog is the animal of choice, since it is easily available and the experimental conditions of maintaining temperature, oxygenation and handling of tissues do not require critically rigid parameters.

These preparations can be stimulated by various types of stimuli thermal, chemical, mechanical and electrical. The electrical stimuli are preferred for experimental studies because: (a) the strength of the stimulus can be precisely controlled, (b) the strength can be easily measured, (c) the tissues respond very precisely, (d) the tissues are not damaged, and (e) the phenomenon of excitation is by itself electrical in nature.

In the description that follows, a brief mention of the equipment and material used is given before describing the dissection and experimental preparations.

AMPHIBIAN RINGER'S SOLUTIONS

To make the isolated or exposed tissues survive for a longer time a solution which is iso-osmotic with the extracellular fluid is necessary. For the frog tissues the amphibian Ringer's solution serves this purpose. It contains NaCl which provides the bulk of its osmolarity. In addition, it contains small amounts of KCl that is necessary for the maintenance of the membrane potential, $CaCl_2$ that is necessary for muscle contraction and $NaHCO_3$ for making the solution weakly alkaline. The composition of the solution is:

NaCl	0.6%
KCl	0.014%
$CaCl_2$	0.012%
$NaHCO_3$	0.02%

Distilled water to 100 ml

Isotonic saline (0.6% NaCl solution) can also be used instead of amphibian Ringer's solution.

1. Kymograph:

- This is the instrument used for recording the contractions of the tissue, i.e., the mechanical events on a moving surface.

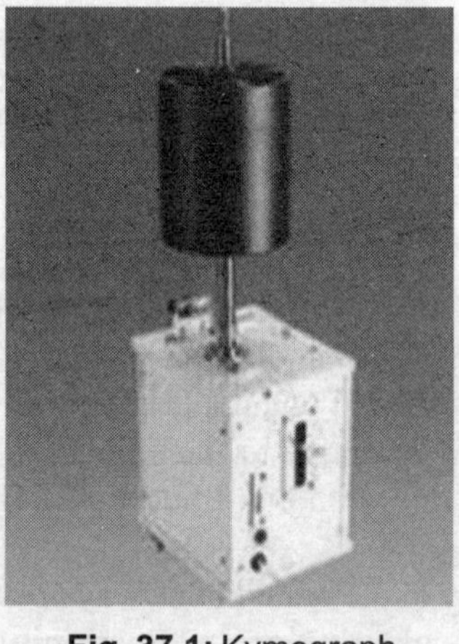

Fig. 37.1: Kymograph

- It consists of a gear-box and a rotating shaft. The cylinder of drum is attached to the rotating shaft. The paper for the recording is pasted on the drum.
- On one side of the gear-box is a speed regulator with the help of which the speed of rotation of the drum can be adjusted.
- On the other side is a switch by which the power supply to the instrument can be switched on or off.
- There is also a clutch for engaging or disengaging the gears.
- Two points for electrical connections with the stimulator are provided on the gear-box. A metal plate is attached to one of these points and it extends up to the second point without touching the latter.
- When this plate is pressed back, it connects both the electrical points. This brought about by a pair of strikers or contact arms provided at the base of the rotating shaft. With the help of this arrangement, the electrical circuit for stimulation can be completed whenever the drum (kymograph) is in circuit.
- Thus, the kymograph has two functions (i) it helps in recording the contractions both points one after other, and (ii) it can also act as a key to make or break the electrical circuit when the drum is included in the circuit.

- **Note:**
  1. If the drum is to be rotated manually disengage the clutch, do not manually rotate the drum when it is in gear and clutch is engaged.
  2. Keep the drum in vertical alignment with the help of the leveling screws provided at the base.

2. **Electrical Stimulator:** This is a step-down transformer having provision for stimulation of biological tissues. The various parts of the stimulator are:

i. *Switch-cum-stimulus mode selector:*
   - When the stimulator is not in use, this is kept in 'off' position.
   - Two switch on the instrument the knob is kept in '*indicator lamb*'.
   - When the drum is needed in circuit, the '*external*' position is used.
   - When single stimulus at a time is to be given, the knob is kept in '*single' position.*
   - When a train of pulses are to be given, the knob is turned to '*Pulse*' position.

ii. *Stimulus out points:* These points are to be connected to the stimulating electrodes.

iii. *Voltage regulator:* With the help of this the strength of the stimulus can be altered.

iv. *Voltage multiplier:* The voltage set by the voltage regulator can be multiplied five times by this.

v. *Drum or external points:* These points are to be connected to the points provided on the gear-box of the kymograph, whenever the drum is included in the circuit.

vi. *Push button:* It is used in 'external' and 'single' positions of the stimulus mode selector.

vii. *Frequency regulator:* With the help of this, the frequency (in cycles per second) of repeated stimulations can be adjusted.

viii. *Width selector:* The duration of the stimulus can be kept at 0.5 or 1.5 msec with this.

3. **Lucas Muscle Trough:** This is a Perspex container in which the isolated nerve-muscle preparation is fixed. Cork pieces are provided in the floor of the container for fixing the tissues. The tissues are covered with Ringer's solution poured into the trough. An outlet for draining off, the Ringer's solution is present at the bottom of the trough. The electrodes and the isotonic lever are to be fixed on this trough. The trough mounted on a stand.

4. **The Electrodes:** Different forms of electrodes are available. The electrodes are connected to the 'stimulus out' points of the stimulator.

5. **Isotonic Lever:** This is fixed to the muscle trough and to one end of it, the pen marker is attached. The muscle is attached to the hook provided in the lever. Whenever the muscle contracts, the hook is pulled forward and the writing point moves up. The lever is also provided with a screw (after loading screw) with the help of which the muscle can be either after-loaded or free-loaded.

6. **Time Marker:** It is an electrical device consisting of a writing point which is made to vibrate at a frequency of 100 cps.

7. **Simple Heart Lever and Starling Heart Lever:** These are the writing levers used to record the contractions of the heart.

8. **Frog Board:** This is a Perspex board, the upper surface of which is covered with cork. It is used in heart experiments, when the entire frog is placed and then fixed to this board. Frog's legs should not be hanging placed and then out and the board is mounted on a stand.

9. **Syme's Cannula:** It is a small glass cannula with a nozzle and a side tube. The side tube is connected by a rubber tube, to a reservoir of Ringer's solution. It is used in the isolated heart perfusion experiments.

ELECTRICAL CONNECTIONS FOR STIMULATION

1. **Drum in Circuit:** In this type of connection, the drum is used as a key to make and break the electrical circuit as in the recording of single muscle twitch and the effect of various stimuli on it (except when demonstrating the genesis of tetanus). For this:
   1. The electrical points on the kymograph are connected to the 'drum' or external points of the stimulator.
   2. Stimulus mode selector is kept in 'external' position.
   3. Voltage regulator is adjusted at a suitable voltage.
   4. The kymograph is rotated and the push button is pressed till a stimulus is delivered to the tissues.
   5. The stimulus is delivered only when the contact arms touch the metal plate on the electrical points of the kymograph and the push button is pressed.
   6. After the recording the point of stimulus can be marked on the graph obtained by manually rotating the drum to the point where the contact drums touch the electrical points on the drum and dropping a line on the graph with the help of the pen marker.
2. **Single Stimulation without the Drum in Circuit:**
   1. Stimulus mode selector is kept in 'single' position.
   2. The voltage regulator is suitably adjusted.
   3. The push button is pressed once.
3. **Repetitive Stimulation:** Repetitive stimulations are used in demonstrating the genesis of tetanus or in vagal stimulation experiments. When repeated stimuli of varying frequencies are to be given the following adjustments are to be made:
   1. The frequency regulator is adjusted to the required frequency. For example, in the stimulation of vagus nerve, a frequency of 20-30 cps is used.
   2. The voltage regulator is suitably adjusted.
   3. Stimulus mode selector is turned to 'Pulses' position.

(**Note:** The push button need not be pushed for repetitive stimulation.)

DISSECTION

Pithing of Frog

- Stun the frog by giving a sharp blow to its head with a heavy object.
- Now hold the stunned frog in the left hand with a piece of a cloth, so that its dorsal surface is towards you, and the ventral surface over your palm and little and ring fingers, and the neck over the middle finger. Use the index finger to hold the frog over its eyes and thumb over the back.
- With the pithing needle, trace in the midline, from above downwards, for a depression, where the skull joins the vertebral column. This can also be known by drawing a transverse imaginary line just behind the external tympanic area and finding out where it cuts the dorsal median line.
- Pass the probe vertically for a short distance. As it touches the spinal cord, there is a sudden jerky movement of the frog.
- From withdraw it to the starting point and turn its direction by 180, i.e., towards the vertebral column to destroy the spinal cord.
- As we proceed, first, there is straightening of legs, followed by loss of tone coincident with the destruction of the spinal cord.
- **Note:** The pithing needle or probe should be round. If flat or rectangular it is difficult to reach the desired length. In case it is difficult to pass the probe through the skin and underlying tissue a small incision can be made with a scalpel prior to insertion.

Dissection for Gastrocnemius-sciatic Preparation

- Cut with a scissors the skin around the middle of frog's trunk and peel off the skin downwards from the legs. Now lay the frog on its ventral side, in the tray.
- Lift the urostyle with the forceps and cut with the scissors on both sides, carefully avoiding any injury to the nerve roots which are immediately underneath it. Snip off the urostyle with the help of a bone cutter.
- Proceed with the dissection along the sides of the vertebral column, separating the sacroiliac joints.
- Cut the vertebral column transversely about three vertebrae above the sacrum.
- Divide the vertebra and the sacrum into two equal parts by bisecting in the midline, avoiding any injury to the sciatic nerve and the nerve roots.
- Trace the sciatic nerve in the thing by separating the muscles on the back of the thigh. The branches of the nerve supplying the muscles in the thigh should be cut and not pulled.
- Separate the tendon of gastrocnemius muscle at the ankle and tie a thread around it. Cut the tendon at its attachment.
- The bone is cut above and below the knee joint, and the muscles of the thigh are also cut just above the knee joint.
- This gives us the gastrocnemius muscle with the knee joint, the sciatic nerve and a part of the vertebral column.

Fixing of the Preparation

- The knee joint is fixed with a pin in the cork at the bottom of the muscle trough, taking care that the nerve is not injured.
- The free end of the thread around the tendon is tied to the hook of the lever.
- A dead-load of 1 gm is added to the lever which keeps the muscle in a slightly stretched state and ensures the lever to return to its original position.
- The position of the lever is adjusted to avoid sagging of the thread and/or overstretching of the muscle.
- The long arm of the lever to which the writing point is attached, should be kept horizontal.
- The muscle-nerve preparation should be kept immersed in Ringer's solution but the electrodes used to stimulate the nerve should never dip into it but the electrodes.

Precautions

a. Nerve should never be stretched.
b. Nerve should not be handled with metallic instruments.
c. Both nerve and muscle should be kept moist with Ringer's solution.

Procedure

- The gastrocnemius-sciatic nerve preparation is dissected out and fixed in the muscle trough.
- Electrical connections are made for 'drum-in-circuit' stimulation.
- Speed of drum is adjusted to 640 mm/s.
- The nerve is gently placed on the stimulating electrodes connected to the electronic stimulator.
- The kymograph is turned on and the tip of the rendering lever is brought in fine contact with the surface of the rotating drum. The line recorded at this stage marks the baseline.
- If a single strong stimulus is delivered now, with the help of the push button, the muscle contracts and gets recorded as the simple muscle twitch (SMT):

1. **Phases of the Simple Muscle Twitch:** After recording the SMT in this way, the latent period (between point of stimulus and initiation of contraction), contraction period (between onset of contraction and peak contraction) and relaxation period (from peak contraction till the end of contraction) are demarcated using curvilinear lines, drawn with the help of the recording lever.

   As the drum speed is known, the duration of the three phases can be calculated.

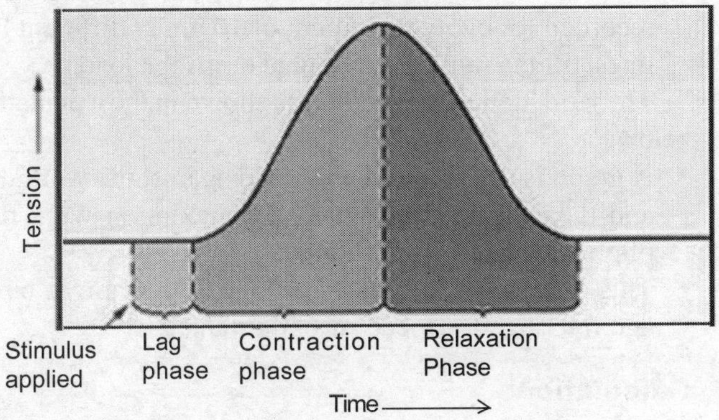

Fig. 37.2

2. Effect of Increasing Strength of Stimulus

- A stimulus of very low strength if first delivered to the muscle. It is noted that no SMT is elicited.
- The strength of stimulus is then gradually increased, allowing at least 3 minutes of interval between stimuli.
- It is noted that it requires a minimal stimulus to trigger an SMT. This strength of stimulus is called the threshold channels while any stress of stimulus less than is called subthreshold and any more than this, suprathreshold.
- With increasing strength of stimulus, its height increases reaching a high limit. The stimulus producing maximum contraction is called the maximal stimulus. Greater stimuli (supramaximal stimuli) fail to increase the strength of the contraction any further. A maximal stimulus stimulates all the muscle fibres in the muscle while submaximal stimuli do not do so.

3. Effect of Temperature on Maximal Contraction

- Even when a maximal stimulus is used, an increase in temperature increases the height of isotonic muscle contraction and reduces the duration of its various phases while a reverse is seen with lower temperature.
- This can be shown by recording at different temperatures (using a ringer solution of say, room temperature, 35°C and 15°C) three SMTs on the same baseline and from the same point of stimulus. Before recording the SMTs, the muscle is allowed to equilibrate thermally for a few minutes with Ringer's solutions at appropriate temperatures.
- Ringer's solution at 42°C or more is not used since the muscle proteins get damaged at those temperatures.
- Determine the height of contraction, latent period, contraction period and relaxation period and tabulate the results in each case.

4. Effect of two Consecutive Maximal Stimuli to Demonstrate Absolute Refractory, Relative Refractory and Beneficial Effect

- Two stimuli can be delivered in quick succession by keeping the drum-in-circuit and using the contact arms on the drum. Take a record as in the case of the simple muscle twitch.
- Open the contact arms of the drum a little and pass the second stimulus in the first half of the latent period. Take the recordings.
- Open the contact arms a little more and pass the second stimulus in second half of latent period and take the recordings.
- In this way by gradually widening the contact arms record the effect of second stimulus given in contraction period, early relaxation, late relaxation period and on completion of the SMT to elicit the beneficial effect.
- The first half of the latent period is on absolute refractory period and the second stimulus is not able to produce an effect. The second half of the latent period onwards is the relative refractory period of the SMT in which there is summation of effects of the stimuli and beneficial effect is seen.

5. Effect of Multiple Maximal Stimuli at High Frequency to Demonstrate the Phenomenon of Tetanus

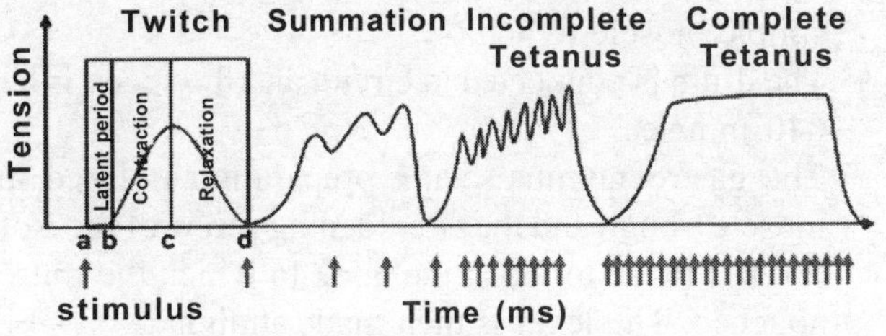

Fig. 37.3

Note:

- The electrical connection for stimulatin are for 'repetitive-stimulations'.
- The kymograph is not in circuit and is adjusted to rotate at a slow speed (12.5 mm/sec).
- The nerve is placed over the electrodes and the strength of the stimulus is so adjusted as to produce a maximal stimulus.
- The frequency of stimulus is adjusted to be at 1 stimulus/sec. The stimulus selector of the stimulator is turned to 'pulses' position. The contractions are on the slow moving drum for a few seconds.
- In the same way the responses are recorded for various frequencies (2, 5, 7, 10, 15, 20, stimuli/sec) till a sustained state of contraction occurs.
- When several consecutive maximal stimuli are delivered at a low frequency, the SMTs recorded are distinct with the lever returning to the baseline between them.
- The first few contractions are of increasing height and have been given the name staircase phenomenon. However, as the frequency of stimulus delivery is increased, the SMTs start fusing together the lever not

returning to the baseline between them. This type of muscle contraction is called incomplete tetanus.

- When the frequency of stimulus deliver is increased further, the serrations produced by the individual SMTs disappear and the tetanus is said to be complete. The strength of tetani contraction is nearly four times that of the SMT.

6. Effect of Load on Muscle Contraction in After Loaded and in Free Loaded Condition

Principle

In after loaded condition the load acts on the muscle during the contraction, i.e., after the onset of contraction and not before the contraction. But in free loaded condition the load acts on the muscle even before the onset of contraction. The load exerts a tension on muscle fibres and the muscle starts the contraction not from a relaxed but from a somewhat stretched state.

PROCEDURE

After Loaded Condition

- The set-up for this experiment is similar to the one for simple muscle twitch.
- The drum is connected in circuit and the speed is kept at 640 mm/sec.
- The gastrocnemius-sciatic preparation is fixed in the muscle trough and the after loading screw of the isotonic lever is made to touch the hook to which the muscle is attached. The lever is then made straight.
- A simple muscle twitch is recorded in the usual manner.
- A 10 gm weight is then attached to the lever with the help of a thread and a twitch is recorded.
- Twitches are recorded in this way for every increment of 10 gm weights till the muscle is not able to lift the load any further.

Note: The strength of stimulus and point of stimulus are not be changed.

Free Loaded Condition

- The drum in this experiment is not in circuit. The clutch is kept in the neutral position as the drum has to be manually moved each time.
- The 'stimulus mode selector' knob of the stimulator is kept at 'single' position.
- The nerve-muscle preparation is fixed in the muscle chamber and the after-loading screw of the lever is released so that the hook of the lever is free to move backwards.
- The lever is made straight, a short base line is recorded by moving the drum manually, the muscle is stimulated and the twitch recorded.
- A 10 gm weight is attached to the lever. As soon as the weight is added, the lever (hence the base-line) moves down. The drum is moved through 1 cm and a twitch is recorded at this point. In this manner, twitches are recorded for every increment of 10 gm at different base lines, till the muscle is not able to lift the load.

The work done is calculated as shown in the calculations below:

- A graph is then plotted with load against the work done and then the load at which the maximum work done (Optimum load) is calculated.
- This experiment can also be done with drum in circuit and moving at a speed of 640 mm/sec.

Calculations

To calculate the work done in each case, the following measurements are taken:

- The height of the contraction : H cm.
- Length of the lever from the fulcrum to the tip: L cm (the long arm of the lever).
- Length of the lever from the fulcrum to the point of attachment of the load (the short arm of the lever): 1 cm.
- The weight or the load lifted : w gm.

The formula for calculating the work done is derived as followed:

Work done = Force acting × Distance through which the force is moved.

= Load added x Distance through which the load is lifted.

= W (cms) × h (cms)

The magnification of the lever : L/I.

The distance 'h' is magnified by L/I times by the lever, to 'H' in the recording. Hence,

$$H = \frac{h \times L}{I}$$

$$h = \frac{H \times I}{L}$$

Hence, the work done : w × h gmcm:

$$\frac{W \times H \times 1 \text{ gm cm}}{L}$$

The figure obtained if multiplied by 981, gives the value in ergs.

A graph is then plotted with load against the work done and then the load at which the maximum work done (Optimum load) is calculated.

Questions:

1. What are the differences in after loading and free loading contractions? Give example of these conditions in the human body.

2. What is the effect of load on the latent period of muscle twitch?
3. Compare the optimum loads in the two conditions.
4. What is the relation between the optimum load and the tension developed in the muscle?

7. Phenomenon of Muscle Fatigue

- Make two gastrocnemius-sciatic preparations and fix one of them in the myograph chamber. Make the connections for the drum in circuit and set the speed of the drum at 640 mm/sec.
- Record a simple muscle twitch as usual and mark the point of stimulus and the point of response.
- Move the lever away from the surface of the drum, set the drum revolving and stimulate the preparation 10 to 15 times. (If the amplitude of contraction has not much changed, stimulate further, till the amplitude visibly decreases).
- Stop the drum and make the lever to touch the surface of the drum as before. Record another simple muscle twitch.
- Repeat this process till the muscle fails to respond.
- Repeated stimulation of the muscle, either directly or through the nerve, causes fatigue, reducing the height of muscle contraction and prolonging all its phases. In addition, the muscle fails to relax completely, which is known as the contraction remainder.

To Demonstrate the Site of Fatigue

- Change the point of stimulus to another portion of the drum.
- Drain off the ringer from the muscle trough.
- Place the electrodes directly on the surface of the muscle and record a base line.
- Now stimulate the muscle and record the response.
- The muscle responds by the contraction and a simple muscle twitch is record. This proves that the muscle is not the site of fatigue.
- Now fix the second gastrocnemius-sciatic preparation in the place of the first one and lay the first preparation by its side.
- Cross the nerves of the two preparations.
- Stimulate the nerve of the first preparation and record the response. The second while keeping the nerve of the first preparation on the electrodes preparation contracts and a simple muscle twitch is recorded. The impulse travels through the nerve of the first preparations, reaches the nerve of the second preparation and stimulates the fresh muscle. This shows that the nerve of the first preparation was also not the site of fatigue.

Questions:

1. Define fatigue.
2. What are the causes of fatigue?
3. Is fatigue a reversible phenomenon?
4. What is contraction remainder?
5. How do you prove that the nerve and muscle are not the sites of fatigue in the above experiment?
6. By what other method you can prove that the nerve is indefatigable?
7. What is the first site of fatigue in an intact animal?
8. What are the conditions that hasten the onset of fatigue?

MEASURING THE SPEED OF NERVE CONDUCTION

For measuring the speed of nerve conduction, two SMTs are recorded: one SMT is recorded by stimulating the nerve at its vertebral end and the other, by stimulating the muscle end of the nerve. The intervening distance between the two electrode position is measured out. The time taken to travel the intervening distance (d cm) results in a difference between the latent periods of the two SMT (t seconds). The speed of nerve conduction will be given by d/t.

Questions:

1. Can a kymograph record bioelectric signals? Give reasons.
2. Which type of muscle contraction has been demonstrated isotonic or isometric?
3. Explain why most of the experiments employ maximal stimuli.
4. Does the skeletal muscle fiber obey the all or none law? Explain.
5. What are the causes for the latent period of a muscle twitch?
6. Recording the contraction and relaxation periods of the muscle twitch helps in classifying skeletal muscles. Explain.
7. Temperature affects isotonic and isometric contraction differently. Explain.
8. Which type of summation has been demonstrated to you: spatial or temporal?
9. Is the summation of muscle contraction associated with the summation of the underlying electrical events? Suggest an experiment that will give an answer to this question.
10. Summation of muscle contraction is observed when the second stimulus falls on the late latent period but not on the early latent period of the first contraction. Explain why.
11. Is their any way of predicting the minimal tetanizing frequency of a muscle? Which is easier to tetanize: red or white skeletal muscle? Can smooth and cardiac muscles be tetanized too?
12. Are voluntary muscle contractions tetanic in nature?
13. Why is a tetanic contraction much greater in strength than a single twitch?

14. Why is a free-loaded muscle contraction greater than an after-loaded contraction even when the loads are equal? Is there an optimal load for a muscle?
15. Why does the contraction remainder occur in a fatigued muscle?
16. What are the possible sites of fatigue in a nerve-muscle preparation? Is the nerve indefatigable? Which is the first site of fatigue in these experiments?